Facial Regeneration Exercises

20 Face Firming Workouts For Men And Women

by Wendy Wilken

Table of Contents

1. SECTION 1

1.1. What This Book Offers You

- Learn 3 face exercises to fade deep forehead and glabellar furrows
- Smooth out craggy crow's feet with these 3 yoga facial exercises
- Dark eye rings can be cured with 4 simple facial exercises
- Significantly diminish ugly eye bags with 4 facial gymnastics workouts
- These 3 face aerobics workouts will help fill out skeletal, hollow eye sockets
- Discover 4 face rubbing exercises to eliminate under eye wrinkles
- Got saggy or chubby cheeks? Apply 3 face toning exercises to firm and lift them
- Perform 3 cheek building exercises to plump up sunken, bony cheeks
- These 3 face rejuvenation exercises reduce face fat and remove mid face plumpness
- Use 5 face regeneration workouts to minimize deep nasal folds and laugh lines
- Discover 3 facial massaging workouts to erase fine mouth and lip lines
- 4 natural facial workouts to tighten and elevate jowls and sagging face skin
- Employ 5 facial firming workouts to drastically reduce a double chin
- Purge wrinkly turkey neck and throat wattle with 3 face toning exercises
- Use 2 neck reshaping exercises to develop and fill out hollow throat regions
- Get a new face glow and healthy skin with 7 facial rubbing exercises
- Learn to merge face yoga and acupressure for permanent age-reversal

1.2. The Advantages Of This Program

- 30 day permanent natural facelift solution – START LOOKING YOUNGER IN DAYS!
- BE THE ENVY of family, friends, and colleagues with your younger, firmer face
- Only 20 quick, easy face exercises to learn and to apply for busy folks, with limited time
- TRIPLE the age-regression benefits by combining face toning and acupressure
- Apply these face exercises for just a few minutes per day, for the first 30 days
- These facial exercises are highly effective for both sexes and all ages - 18 to 85 years old
- 21 little-known secrets and hints to FAST-TRACK your face workout RESULTS
- A shorter version included - just 10 face exercises for people pressed for time
- NO page fillers or unnecessary waffle – Wendy gets to the point quickly
- NO tugging or pulling of facial skin which could unintentionally worsen wrinkles
- NO pulling of weird expressions like other face yoga programs
- NO complicated face exercises as in most face workout regimes
- NO isometrics involved – Only simple facial toning and acupressure methods are used

1.3. About The Author And This Book

Wendy Wilken is a physiotherapist and world-renown facial exercise practitioner.

Wendy Wilken presents her unique facial exercise program, which demonstrates how to practice face and neck toning workouts on targeted acupressure points. The goal of these regimens is to reverse the aging process completely naturally, with little effort, and for huge rewards.

Crisp black-and-white photographs illustrate exactly where to locate the 20 exercise points, on the face and neck. Accompanying narrations explain how to find them, and clearly describe how to perform the facial toning techniques on each spot - with the benefits of that face exercise. One minute of massage on each point, repeated a few times a week, is all it takes to HALT AND REVERSE THE SIGNS OF AGING!

Once you start the program, you will notice that after a few days, your skin will boast new flush and color, be firmer and lifted, and wrinkles will be shallower. The more time and effort you put in, the better the results. Improved circulation will revive once blood-starved skin, tissue, and underlying muscles.

Wendy's non-surgical facelift exercise system employs facial rubbing regimens, using the fingertips on acupressure nodal points. This combination TURBO-BOOSTS YOUR FACE TONING EFFORTS THREE-FOLD.

Facial Regeneration Exercises differs from other face yoga programs, because most are based on radical skin stretching and isometrics, which entail the pulling of weird expressions. THIS PROGRAM DOES NOT INVOLVE STRETCHING THE SKIN OR MAKING WEIRD FACES. Wendy's system is based on gentle exercising of the tissue beneath the skin, using your fingers, thereby TIGHTENING SLACK SKIN FOR A SMOOTH AND YOUNGER LOOK - in a short time period.

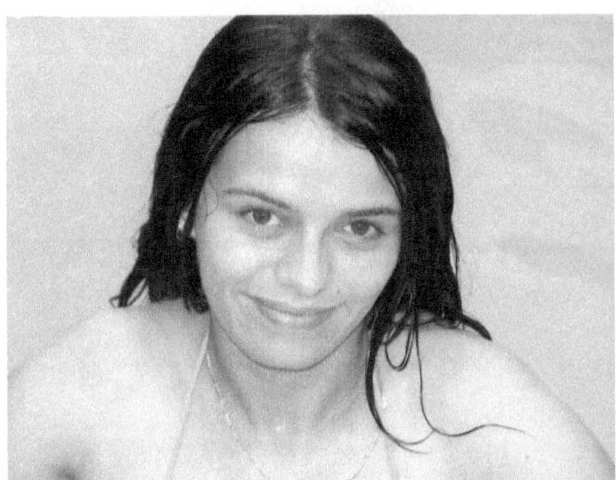

Wendy Wilken – Creator And Author Of The "Facial Regeneration Exercises" Program

2. SECTION 2
2.1. Welcome To Regaining Your Youth!

Thank you for purchasing this book. I am sure that the facial exercise regimens demonstrated in this program will benefit you in many ways, as it has me over the years. In this program, I will cover everything you need to know on how to look years younger, in a relatively short period of time, using facial exercises on acupressure nodal points. Your fingertips are the main tools that you will employ. The principles portrayed here incorporate both acupressure and tissue toning techniques.

My name is Wendy Wilken. I have written this book because I am very passionate about this little-known subject, and love the amazing results it has bestowed on tens of thousands of men and women, worldwide.

Please read it cover-to-cover before starting, as this will give you a good idea how your non-surgical facelift comes together. It should take you about half an hour to read the entire program. I have deliberately made it concise, so that all the important stuff can be conveyed to you - without unnecessary waffle that takes up your precious time! The skin tips and supplementary information are just as important as the step-by-step 20 point face exercise regimens, to attain a perfect non-invasive facelift.

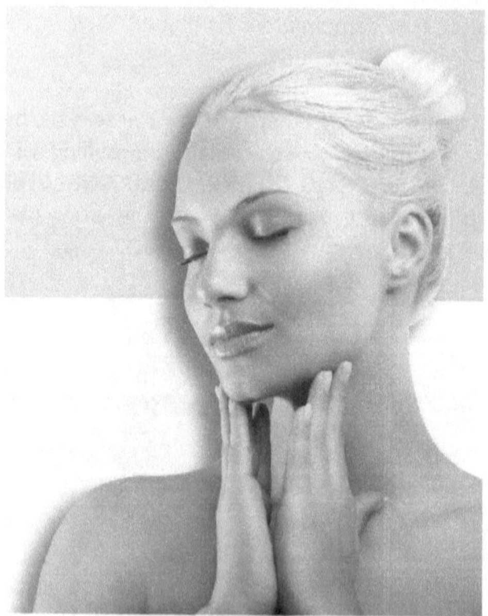

2.2. The Principles Behind Facial Exercises

There are 2 primary types of face exercises that are popular today:

1. Face yoga, using isometrics, which entails the stretching of muscle and skin as an exercising technique.

2. Facial toning workouts, using mostly the fingertips, which exercise the underlying muscles, tissue, and skin.

Facial Regeneration Exercises employs the latter technique, which is muscle and skin toning to tighten baggy skin, and smooth out wrinkles.

Let's explain how these face exercise routines work, without getting too technical:

There are more than 50 muscles in the face and neck. When you stimulate the tissue and muscle, blood flow is increased, and the muscle fiber expands. Increased blood flow to tissue and skin means that the cells which were once starved, are now nourished. Blood brings essential nutrients to the skin, thereby rejuvenating it, and giving it the ability to heal. Collagen manufacture increases, and consequently, so does the skin's elasticity. This all helps to combat and eradicate wrinkles, creases, and folds.

As you know, muscle lies between bone and the skin. When you exercise the muscle, it expands. This expansion and muscle strengthening pulls the skin towards it, which means that the skin gets tighter and more shapely, much like the rippling of muscle on a fit person's stomach!

Now that the skin is pulled taut - lines, furrows, indentations, and even acne scars - become shallower, with regular face exercise routines. Renewed color makes you look younger and more vital. Once commencing the workouts in this program, your facial transformation will occur in front of your eyes - over a period of days, weeks, and months!

2.3. The Combination Of Facial Exercises Applied On Acupressure Points

Acupressure has been around for thousands of years, and is just as effective as acupuncture. The ancient Chinese discovered that the body comprises a series of intricate energy lines (meridians), and energy points (nodal points), which rest on these lines. Each nodal point corresponds to an organ, body part, or treats a specific health element, when stimulated. Manipulating these nodal points with needles (acupuncture) treats certain ailments, and improves conditions in the body and can rejuvenate the skin.

Acupressure, which encompasses massaging with one's own thumbs or fingertips, helps to open the energy channels in the nodal points and meridians. This energy flow is often called *Chi* in Chinese, and *Ki* in Japanese. These techniques harmonize the body's natural energy and rhythm, thereby resulting in better overall health. By performing acupressure on the face and neck on specific nodal points, this enhances blood circulation and *Chi* to the face and neck, which rejuvenates the cells in the epidermis and the underlying tissue and muscle. Acupressure, practiced on certain points on the face, significantly boosts anti-aging efforts and general health, and makes you look younger with regular massage.

Acupressure and facial exercises by themselves, are a powerful weapon against baggy skin, lines, and aging symptoms. The secret to this program is COMBINING THESE TWO SUPER WEAPONS to create an unstoppable force - that systematically chips away at the symptoms of aging, over a period of time. Face workouts, performed on the acupressure nodal points, enhance the benefits threefold, as opposed to facial exercises on their own.

Success depends on how much dedication, time, and effort you put into face workouts. This facial rejuvenation methodology should become a way of life for you, much like eating and bathing, to be really effective over the long term. You do not have to spend much time doing the face exercises, but frequency of doing the regimens is important. What effort you put in, you will get out - in the form of age-regression benefits. This is the life-changing legacy that the Facial Regeneration Exercises program will bring to your life!

Please note: You cannot restructure natural face bone structure. However, you can reshape and work tissue and muscle fiber that rest on the bone, for facial improvement. The regimens in this book will help you to radically improve your looks, smooth out wrinkles, lift and tighten sagging skin that mars your appearance, and reverse the signs of aging.

Just in case you were wondering, I was 29 years old when these photographs were taken and this program was compiled. I never wear makeup, because I have nothing to hide - due to this program's age-regression attributes. I started applying these face exercise regimens when I was 20 years old, and the results yielded over the 9 years(when the photographs in this book were taken), are testament to the success of the combination of these face exercises and acupressure routines.

My picture is at the beginning of this book, and I am the person demonstrating the face workout points and facial exercise routines in all the black-and-white pictures in this book.

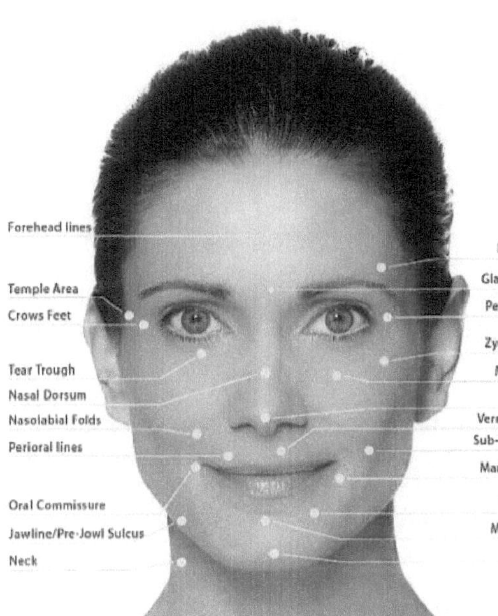

Forehead lines
Lateral Brow
Glabellar Region
Temple Area
Periorbital Area
Crows Feet
Zygomatic Arch
Tear Trough
Malar Region
Nasal Dorsum
Nasal Tip
Nasolabial Folds
Vermillion Border
Perioral lines
Sub-malar Region
Marionette Lines
Oral Commissure
Lateral Chin
Jawline/Pre-Jowl Sulcus
Mental Crease
Neck
Chin

2.4. Facial Exercises And The Time Factor

People frequently ask me in what time period they will notice results, after starting the techniques in this program - such as, when their complexion begins to flush with color, the skin tightens, and wrinkles fade. The answer is this: It depends on many factors - such as age, sex, and health of the patient, skin type, genetics, sun and free radical damage, smoking, old scarring, previous invasive cosmetic procedures undertaken, dedication and effort put into the regimens, and many others. These are all elements that can determine the extent of benefits one will derive from this program, in a given time frame.

There are many women and men in their late 40's and early 50's that have lost 10 to 15 years off their looks, in the first 30 days of commencing this program. And there are those folk where it takes a little longer. The extent of success depends on the factors described above. Often, there are parts of the face and neck that improve relatively easily within a short period, and there are some facial regions that take more time and effort. My suggestion is to go back to those regions of the face that need attention, and spend more time on them immediately after completing the basic 20 point set, as described later in this book.

To a large degree, the face exercise success formula can simply be written down as:

Effort Put Into The Face Exercises + Time Taken Doing The Exercises = Excellent Results

This means that you need to adhere to the 20 point regimens regularly, and do them over a period of time to yield the age-regression benefits you seek. Reason and reality needs to be taken into consideration too; you cannot be 25 years of age and expect to lose 10 years off your looks to appear 15 years old again. It is just not possible! Likewise, it is not conceivable to be 60 years of age and expect to look 25 again, within 30 days of commencing these facial exercises!

These methods are a process - that involves patience, time, and just a little effort. As the days, weeks, and months pass you WILL reap great results! Your non-invasive facelift is literally at your fingertips, and under your control.

The sooner you start the 20 point system in life, the better - simply because these face exercises thwart free radical damage, and repair cellular breakdown that has occurred over the years. Regular face exercising will maintain healthy blood circulation through the capillaries in the skin, and keep the energy channels open. Remember, whatever wrinkles and sagging skin you possess now, have taken a lifetime to manifest. One cannot expect these to disappear overnight. Sticking to the regimens will at first halt the decay of your looks, and then start to reverse the symptoms of aging. Wrinkles WILL fade and disappear, baggy and wrinkly skin WILL tighten over time. Give these face workouts their due, and the rewards you shall reap will be bountiful and awesome! It is never too early or too late to start, even if you are in your 60's, 70's or 80's.

2.5. The Benefits Of Facial Exercises And Face Acupressure Toning

Using the principles laid out in this book, over a period of time, will yield you the following benefits:

1. You will look younger.

2. Wrinkles will smooth out, crinkly and saggy skin will become firm, eye bags and dark circles will fade.

3. Skin texture, tone, and color will improve and appear fresher. Collagen manufacture will be boosted, and skin elasticity will be restored somewhat.

4. Hollow areas such as gaunt cheeks, eye sockets, and skinny neck will fill and inflate. On the other hand, double chin, chubby cheeks will become leaner and more chiseled.

5. Certain ancillary health benefits can be derived - such as improved digestion, better sleep, relief from migraines and headaches. You will experience more harmony with your body.

6. Face exercises are free of charge, and offer you the ability to achieve your own non-surgical facelift - without cost, pain, risk, and inconvenience.

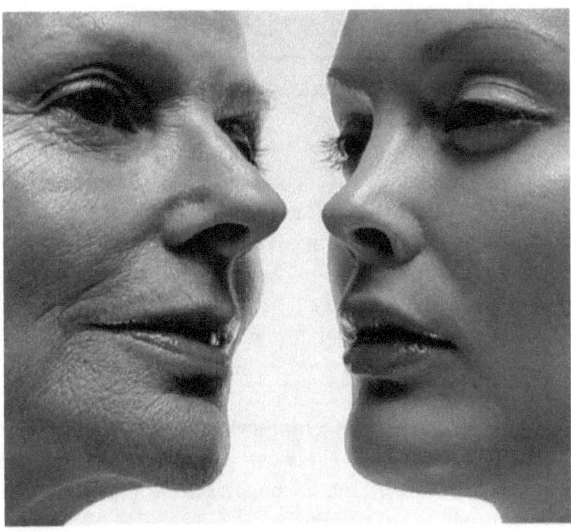

2.6. How To Perform Your Facial Exercises With Ease

Here are some pointers to note before you start the program:

1. For the first 30 days, please conduct the 20 point program every day. Try not to skip a day. Regularity of the face workouts will open the energy channels, and improve blood circulation to and from the acupressure points.

2. After exercising the 20 points, you can return to problem areas such as sagging jowls, hollow cheeks, frown lines, etc. You do not have to do this if you do not have the time, but it is highly recommended.

3. After the first month, you may still perform the regimens daily, but you will find that you can probably maintain your facelift by doing the routines 2-3 times a week. When I say maintain, I mean either sustain your progress so far, and/or gradually improve your results after the first 30 days. The more effort you put into your regimens, the sooner you will appear younger, and the more effective the routines will be.

4. Try to perform the regimens while listening to soothing background music, which will relieve you of any stress and help you to relax while you conduct the massaging. Or, practice them with whatever chills you out, such as watching television.

5. You can do them any time of the day or night. I prefer to conduct these face exercises at night, because the pressures of the day are behind me, and I am in a more relaxed state. If time constraints are a problem, then you can perform them literally anywhere, such as at the bus stop, in traffic, at the office, etc.

6. You might have printed this book out, or saved it on your iPad or Kindle for quick access. Place the book in front of you (in whatever format), and flip to "Facial Exercise Point 1". Follow the instructions as per the narration, and mimic the photo illustration to locate the massage point. Exercise as directed. Then move to "Facial Exercise Point 2", and so on, until you have completed all 20 points. After a few days, you will not even need to consult the book any longer, as you should by then know all the points without having to refer to the illustrations.

7. It is to your advantage to apply the techniques from the top of your face, and work your way downwards, as directed. This will boost your face exercise regimens and eliminate wrinkles, lines, and creases faster, and lift baggy skin. Energy flow and blood circulation to the skin and tissue cells will be maximized.

8. Avoid massaging any area that is wounded, bruised, cut, or damaged until it is completely healed.

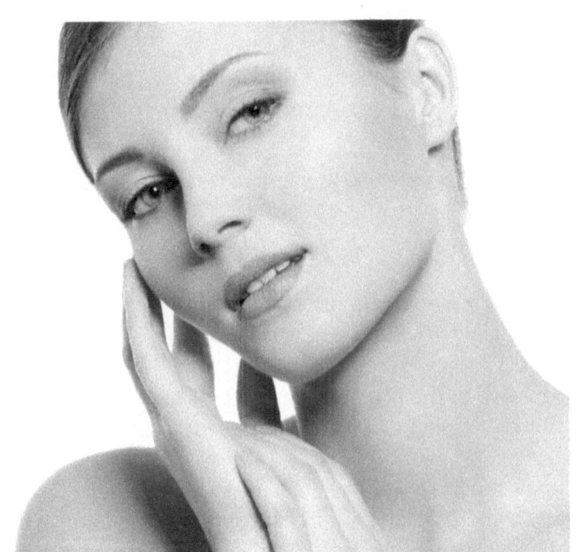

2.7. How To Locate The Acupressure Points

1. Sit in front of a full mirror, where you are able to clearly see your face and neck.

2. Relax your body, especially your neck and shoulders.

3. Position this book in a place where you can view it in paper form, or iPad/Kindle format. Refer to the section called "The 20 Point Facial Exercise Program With Pictures, Directions, And Descriptions" at "Facial Exercise Point 1". Carefully read the narration as to how to position your fingertips on the acupressure points. Look at the picture that corresponds to the points, and then verify that you have them correct in the mirror.

4. You will find a small depression at each acupressure nodal point. With your fingertips, use firm pressure (not too hard so that it hurts or causes discomfort), and practice the massage as indicated by the illustrations and narratives. Some of the motions are done with thumbs, some with forefingers, and one with the back of the hand (or hands). Some motions are circular i.e. inward or outward; some demand a clockwise or anticlockwise movement. Follow the directions in the program to the best of your ability, for maximum results. Do not get frustrated if you are not sure whether you have located the exact acupressure points. As long as you are in the near vicinity, your facial exercises will work their magic! Likewise, it is not too important if you conduct inward or outward motions with your fingertips, or perform them clockwise or anticlockwise. The important thing is that you do the face and neck workouts to the best of your ability, and as close to the directions of this book as you can.

5. Massage each acupressure point for AT LEAST ONE MINUTE, but not more than four minutes at a time. Performing a facial workout on one spot for longer in one go is overdoing it, and thus counter-productive. Clock the face exercises if you wish, but do not stress about exact timing. You can always go back to the same points later in the day, or after your basic 20 point set, if you wish. Go through the facial exercise regimens, working from the top (the forehead) to bottom, and preferably in the given order at your own relaxed pace, and you will soon be executing the entire program at a smooth, comfortable pace.

6. If the points are symmetrically on either side of your face, massage them simultaneously, as guided by this book.

7. Do not push your face into the fingers, otherwise you might suffer from a stiff neck or shoulders. Keep your face vertical, unless directed otherwise, and push your fingers into the tissue. Not too hard, though!

8. When massaging with the forefingers or thumbs, press into the underlying tissue so that it shifts under the skin. The aim is to stimulate the muscle and tissue BENEATH the skin, without necessarily stretching the skin. The skin should move slightly with the muscle tissue as you exercise - without overly stretching it.

9. Inhale and exhale slowly and deeply through your mouth while performing the face workouts. This will enhance oxygen supply throughout your body, muscles, tissue, and skin cells, and help you to expel toxins from your lungs.

10. Some folks might experience a pleasant tingly sensation in certain zones on the face and neck, when they exercise. This is a good indication that the energy points are optimally open, and that the blood is flowing unrestricted to your muscles, tissue, and skin. Do not worry if you do not experience this; you will still receive your age-regression benefits, as long as you do the face workouts regularly and thoroughly.

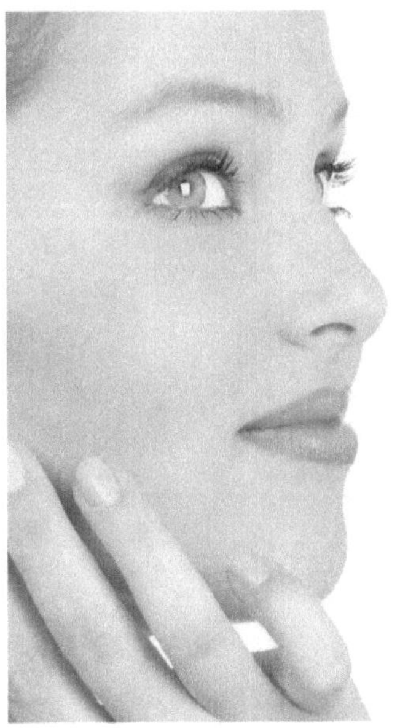

3. SECTION 3
3.1. The 20 Point Facial Exercise Program With Pictures, Directions, Descriptions

We now get to the actual face exercises themselves, practicing them in the sequence that you should perform them. Notice, that we start at the top, and work our way downwards.

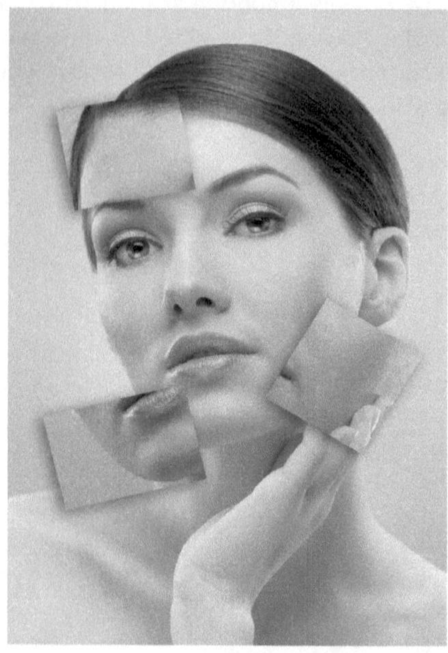

3.1.1. Facial Exercise Point 1

Location: On the hairline, just above your eyes and in line with the pupils.

Motion: Practice small inward circles, using firm pressure with both forefingers, for at least one minute.

Primary Target: Forehead lines, sagging face skin

Benefit: This face exercise tackles forehead furrows and lines, and opens the flow of energy down into your face. The thin muscles in this area will be relaxed and invigorated by the action of the massage.

Oriental Acupressure Name: *Mei Jung*

Other Effects: You might experience some pleasant feelings in your abdomen whilst doing this massage. This acupressure point is on the meridian line which regulates the gall bladder and liver. This regimen also treats mild to severe headaches.

3.1.1.1. Point 1 Front View

Point 1 Front View

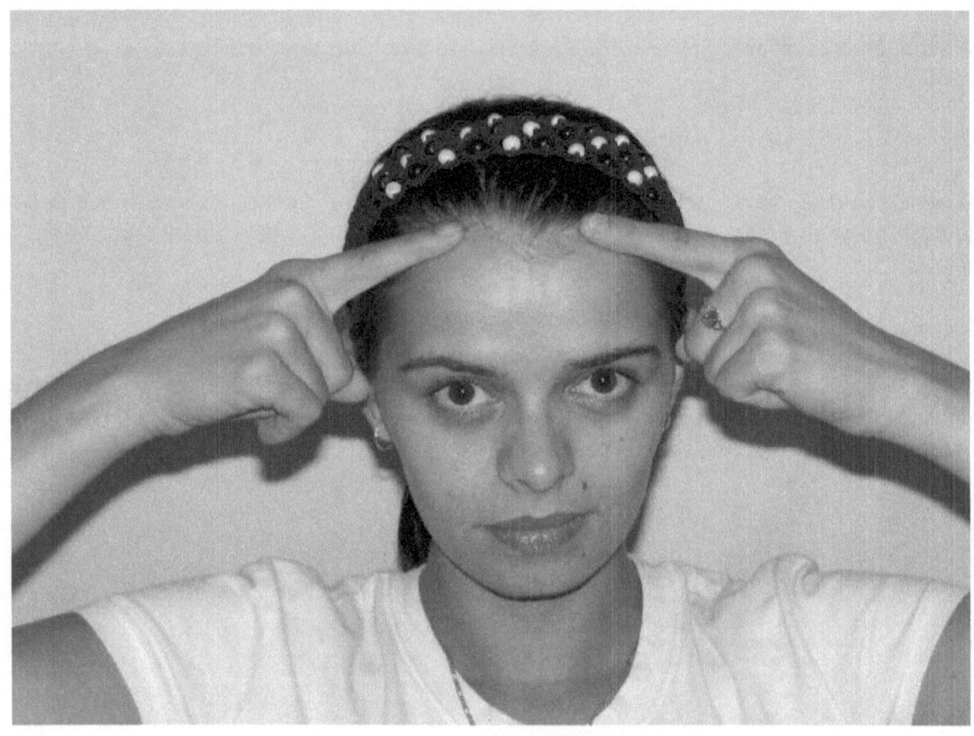

3.1.1.2. Point 1 Side View

Point 1 Side View

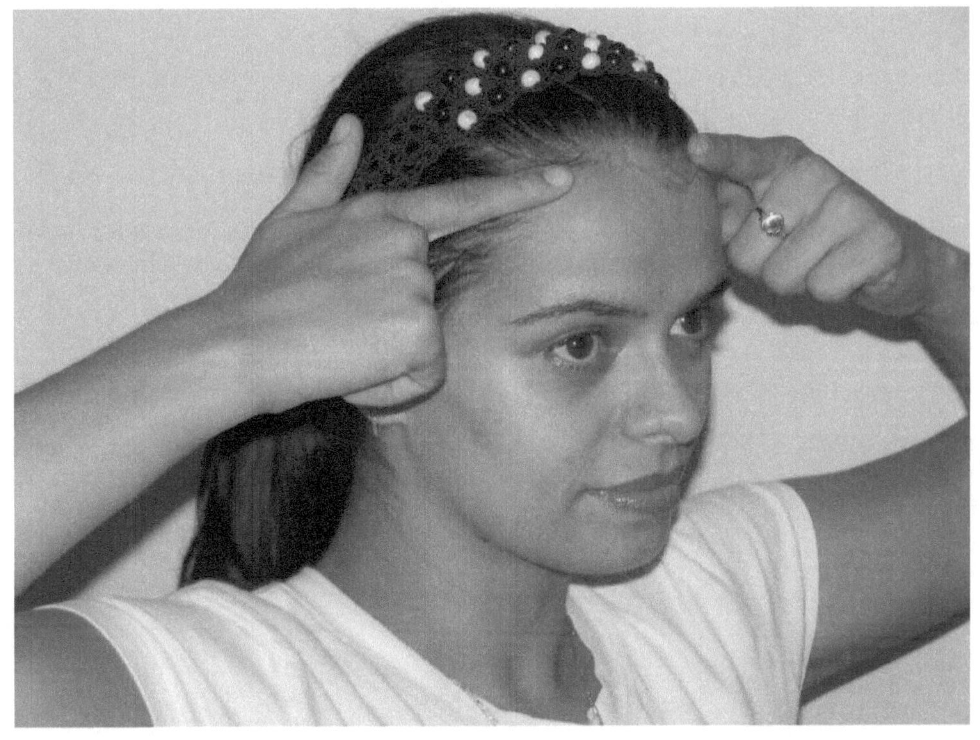

3.1.2. Facial Exercise Point 2

Location: Below the previous point, midway between the hairline and the top of the eyebrows, in line with the pupils.

Motion: Practice small inward circles, using firm pressure with both forefingers, for at least one minute.

Primary Target: Forehead lines, sagging face skin, refresh skin color and glow

Benefit: Massaging these points works on the skin and the forehead muscles, which support the layers of skin which have a tendency to develop deep wrinkles - due to facial expressions and free radicals. This facelift exercise will help stimulate and build up the underlying muscle tissue for a smooth brow.

Oriental Acupressure Name: *Yang Bai*

Other Effects: Massaging this point is very soothing. You may feel some warmth on the face and the back of the neck. This acupressure point also treats migraine headaches and insomnia.

3.1.2.1. Point 2 Front View

Point 2 Front View

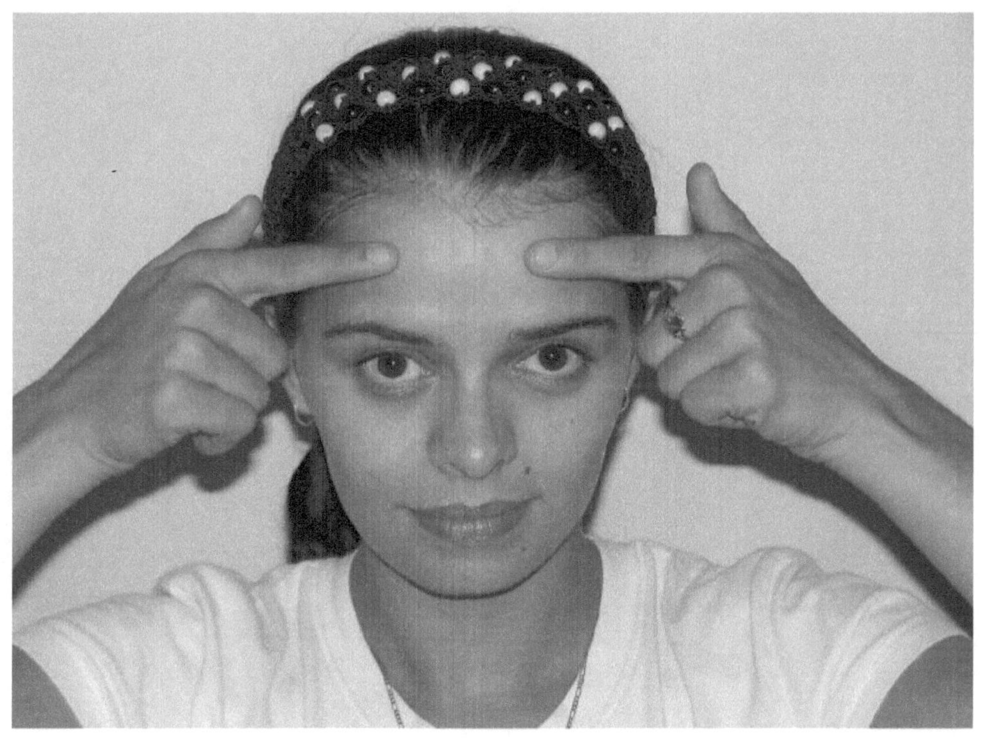

3.1.2.2. Point 2 Side View

Point 2 Side View

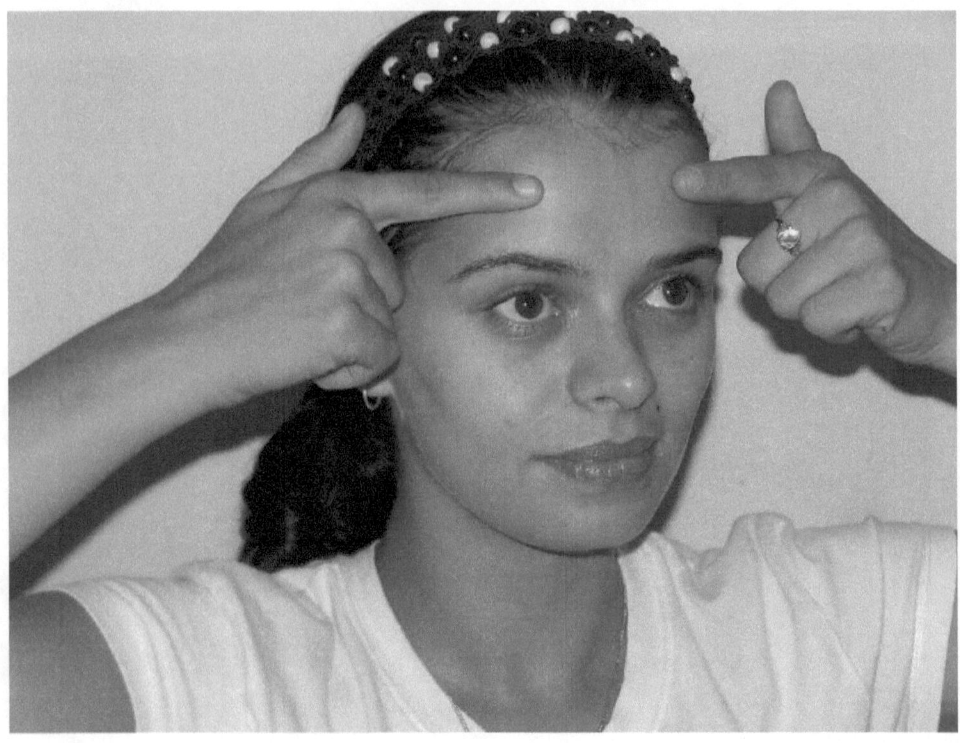

3.1.3. Facial Exercise Point 3

Location: Between the eyebrows, above the bridge of the nose.

Motion: Practice small inward circles using firm pressure with your right forefinger, for at least one minute.

Primary Target: Worry lines, forehead creases

Benefit: This face exercise prevents, softens, and fades vertical frown lines situated between the eyebrows, and on the lower forehead area.

Oriental Acupressure Name: *Yintang*

Other Effects: Massaging here treats headaches, and can also improve stomach and liver function. It also channels energy to the middle and lower face.

3.1.3.1. Point 3 Front View

Point 3 Front View

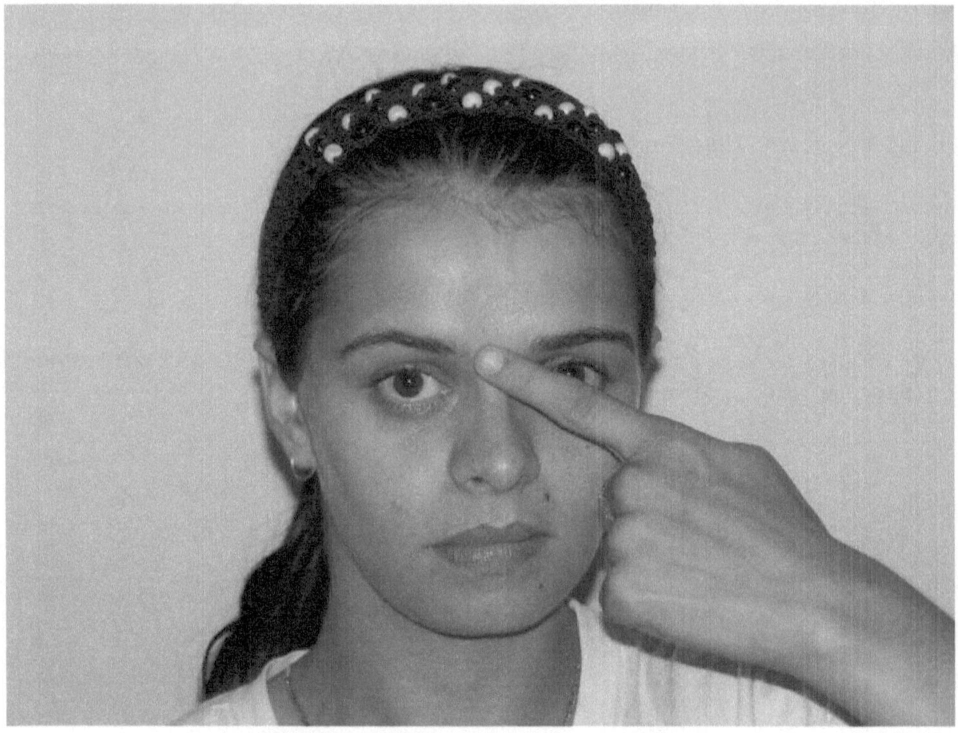

3.1.3.2. Point 3 Side View

Point 3 Side View

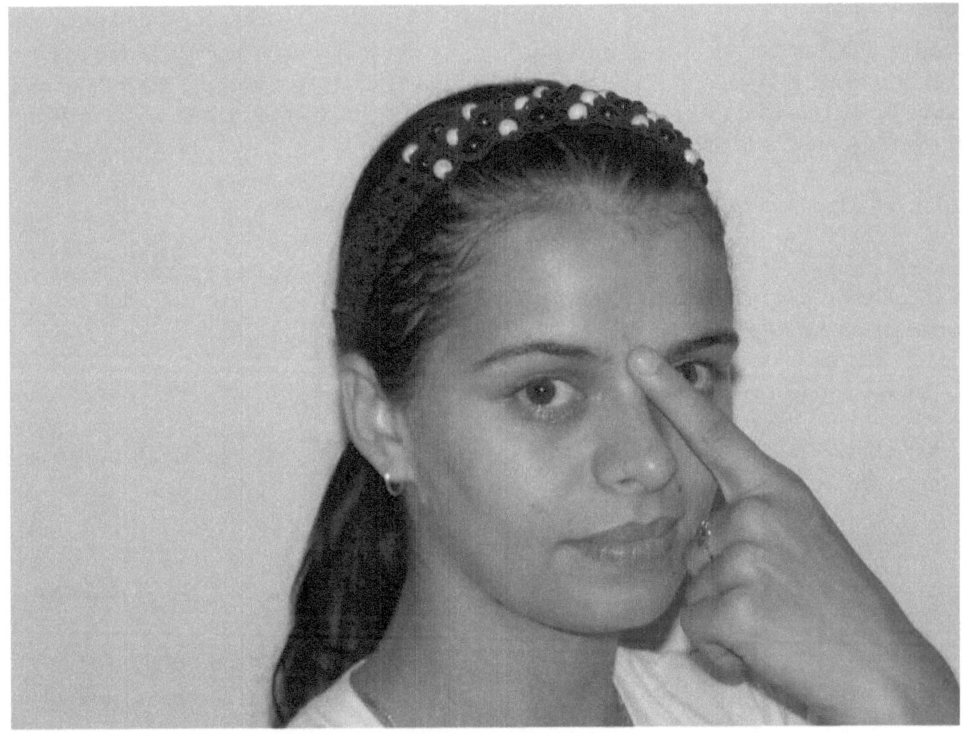

3.1.4. Facial Exercise Point 4

Location: On the inside of your eye sockets, on either side of the bridge of the nose.

Motion: Use your thumbs instead of your fingertips. Place your thumbs against each side of the top part of the bridge of your nose, and rotate upwards just under the eyebrows. The thumbs must fit perfectly into the contour of the inside corner of the eyes, in the eye sockets. Make small inward circles for at least one minute, without pushing into the eyes.

Primary Target: Dark circles, eye wrinkles, eye bags, under eye wrinkles

Benefit: By massaging this area, you will stimulate the flow of energy down around the eyes, nose, and center of the face. This facial exercise will improve dark circles, eye bags, and frown lines between the eyebrows.

Oriental Acupressure Name: *Zan Zhu*

Other Effects: This massage technique is sometimes used to treat headaches, eyestrain, and general eye discomfort. It is also used to relieve sinus tension.

3.1.4.1. Point 4 Front View

Point 4 Front View

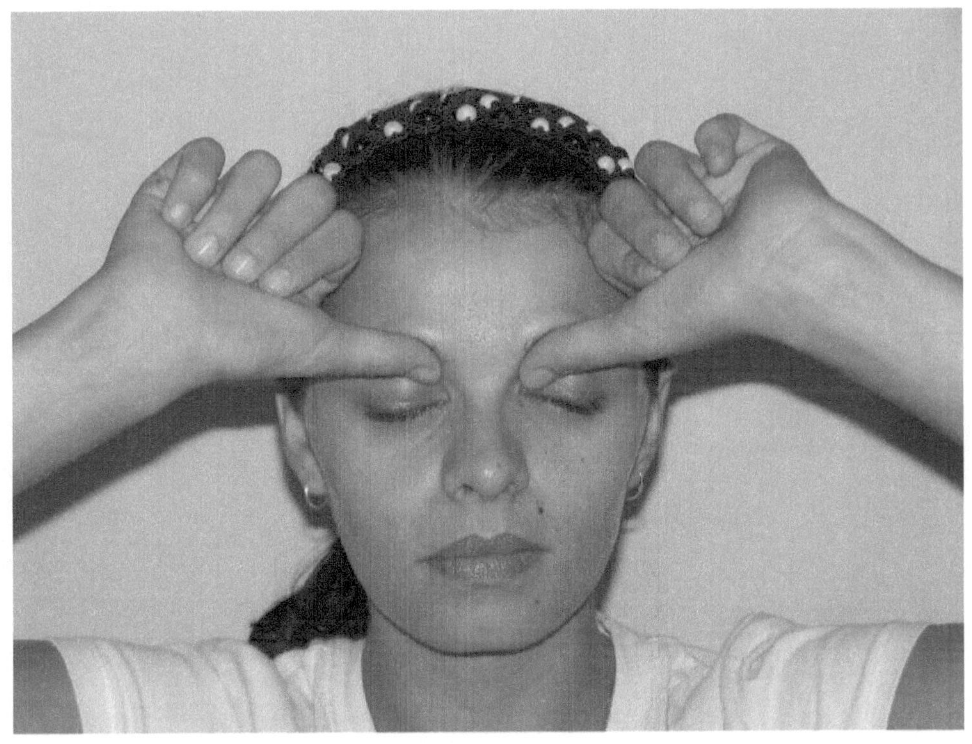

3.1.4.2. Point 4 Side View

Point 4 Side View

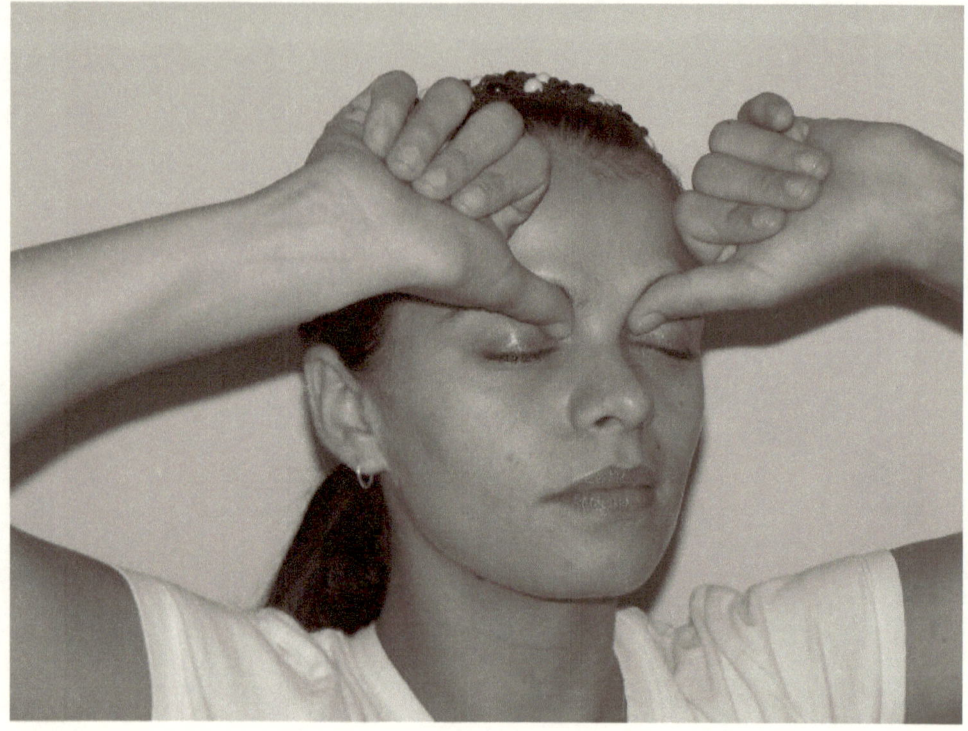

3.1.5. Facial Exercise Point 5

Location: At the far ends of the eyebrows.

Motion: Practice small outward circles using firm pressure with your forefingers. Breathe easily, and relax any tension you may have in your neck and shoulders, while performing this technique. Close your eyes if necessary. Do this face workout for at least one minute.

Primary Target: Crow's feet, eye wrinkles, dark circles, eye bags, under eye wrinkles

Benefit: This point works on the delicate muscle structure above the eyes and temples. It stimulates the underlying muscles, and revives them. This is one of the points that are beneficial to fade crow's feet and eye wrinkles, as it helps to expand the tissue under the creases.

Oriental Acupressure Name: *Sizhu Kong*

Other Effects: This also helps with the treatment of headaches.

3.1.5.1. Point 5 Front View

Point 5 Front View

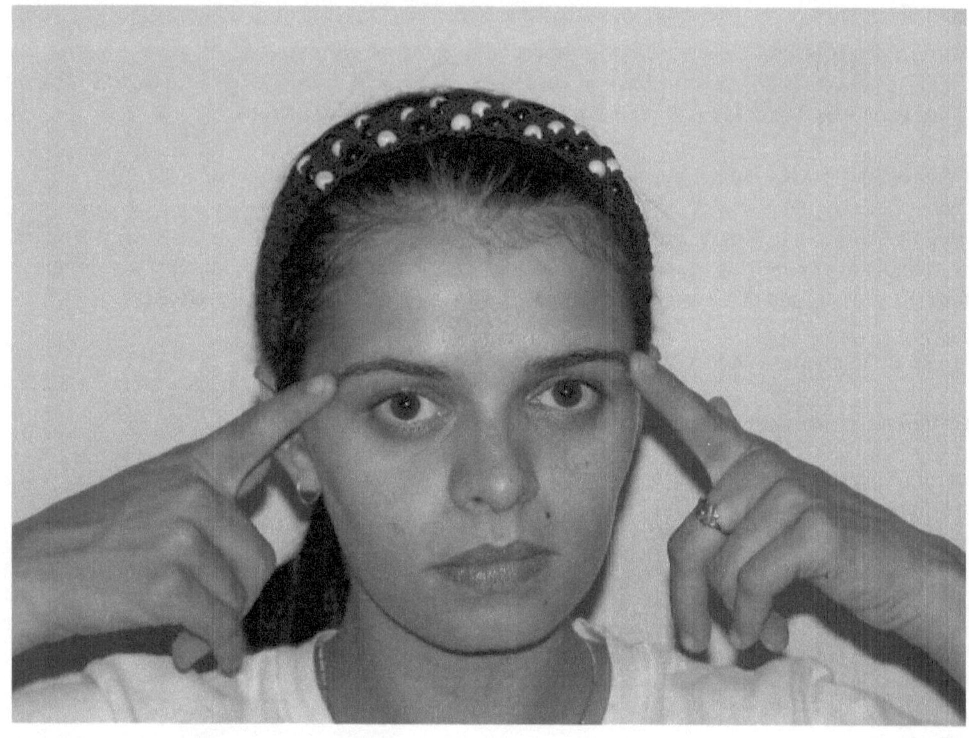

3.1.5.2. Point 5 Side View

Point 5 Side View

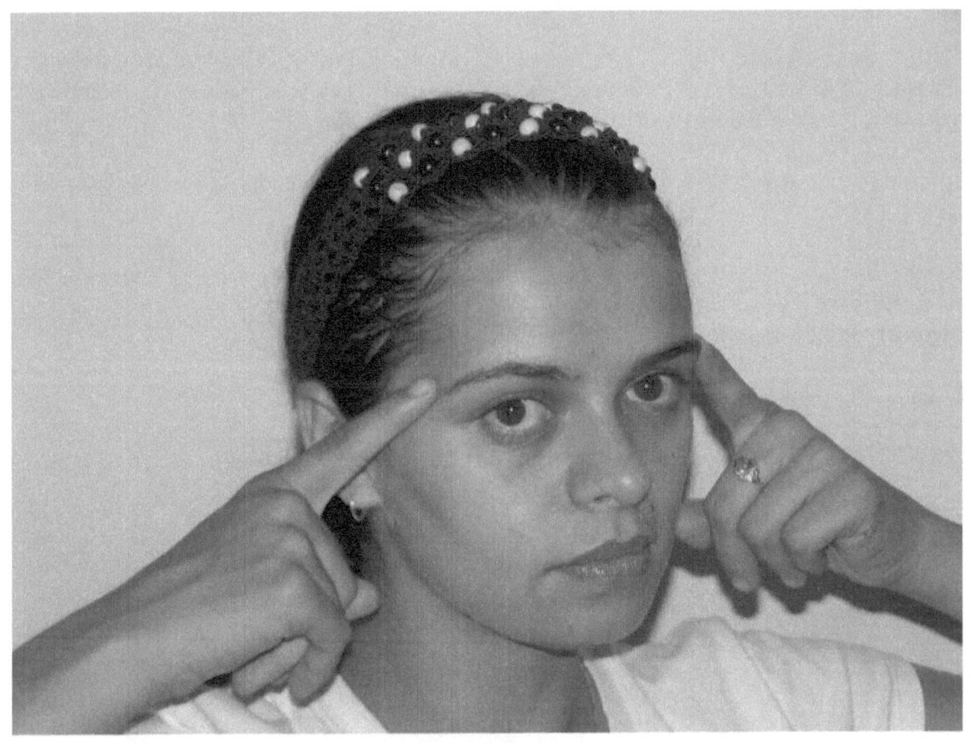

3.1.6. Facial Exercise Point 6

Location: At the outside corner of the eyes, where the crow's feet are located.

Motion: Do small outward circles in the depression of the muscle, using firm pressure with your fingertips. Avoid pushing against the eyeballs. You may leave your eyes open or closed while massaging this point. Exercise for at least one minute on this spot.

Primary Target: Crow's feet, eye wrinkles, dark circles, eye bags, under eye wrinkles, sunken eye sockets

Benefit: This face exercise enhances blood circulation to the eye area and treats crow's feet, squint lines, eye bags, and dark rings. The small muscles become energized and toned, whilst the skin becomes supple and softer.

Oriental Acupressure Name: *Wai Ming*

Other Effects: This workout can alleviate irritated or dry eye syndrome.

3.1.6.1. Point 6 Front View

Point 6 Front View

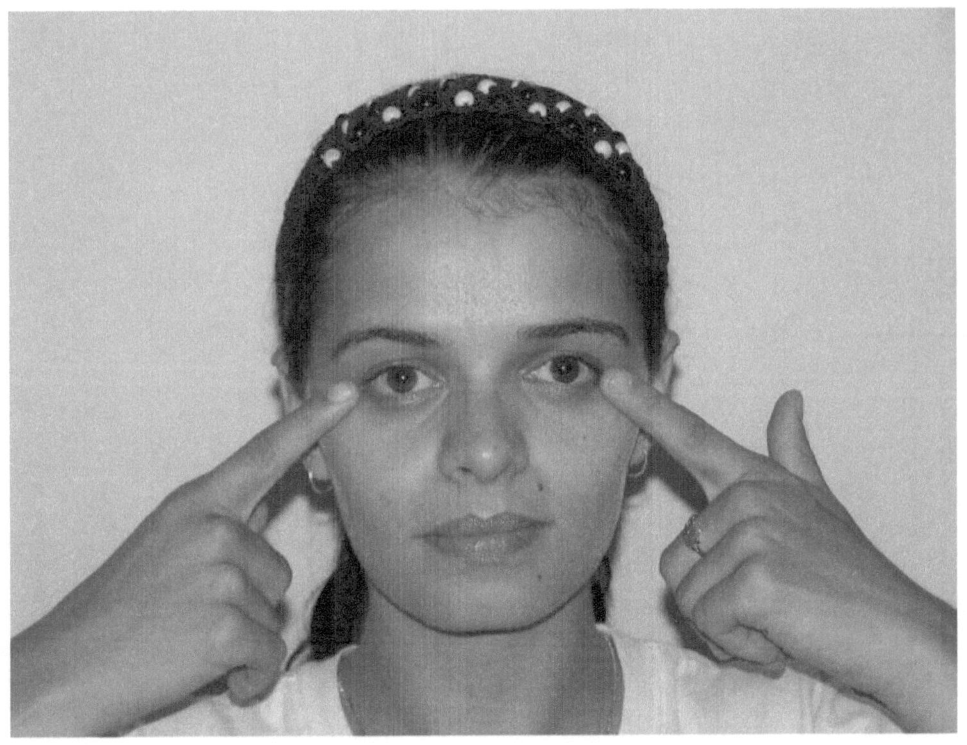

3.1.6.2. Point 6 Side View

Point 6 Side View

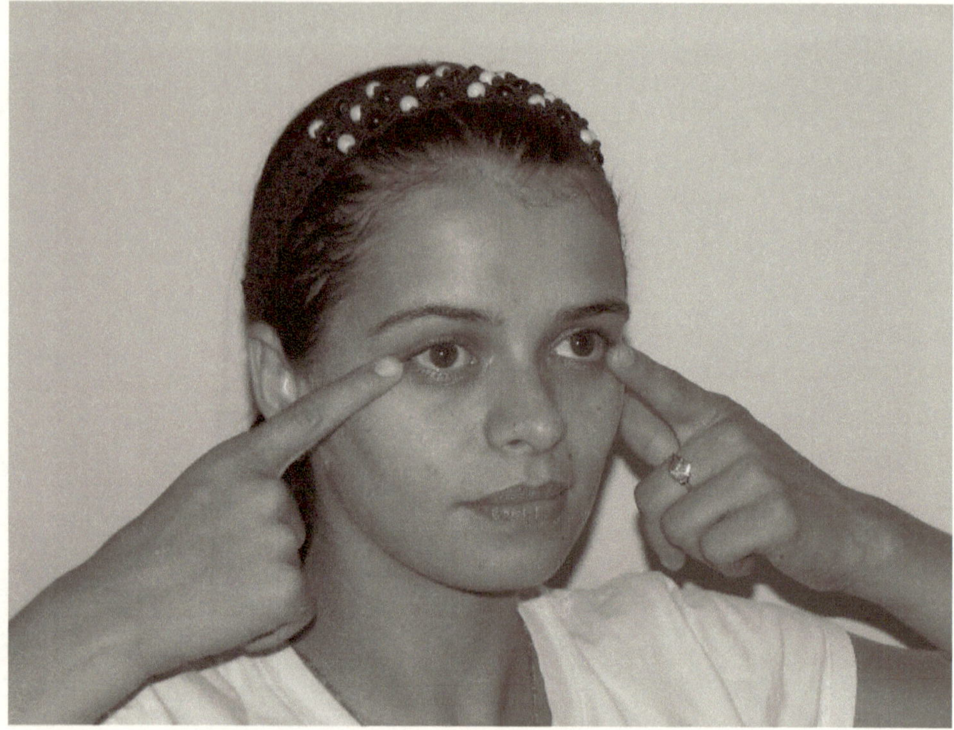

3.1.7. Facial Exercise Point 7

Location: On the edge of the eye sockets, directly below, and in line with the pupils.

Motion: With the forefingers, make small outward circles in the curve of the lower eye sockets. The correct spot is on the bone where eye bags are present, or are most likely to form. Do this exercise for at least one minute. Again, be careful not to push against the eyeballs. It is preferable that you leave your eyes open while massaging this point.

Primary Target: Eye bags, under eye wrinkles, dark circles, crow's feet, chubby cheeks, hollow cheeks, sunken eye sockets, refresh skin color and glow

Benefit: This facial workout enhances blood circulation in the local eye tissue, thereby improving the skin condition in this area. Dark eye circles, bags under the eyes, and under eye wrinkles will become less pronounced, and will fade. The fatty deposits that accumulate under the eyes will also dissipate over time.

Oriental Acupressure Name: *Cheng Qi*

Other Effects: This technique can relieve eyestrain and stress-related tension around the eyes.

3.1.7.1. Point 7 Front View

Point 7 Front View

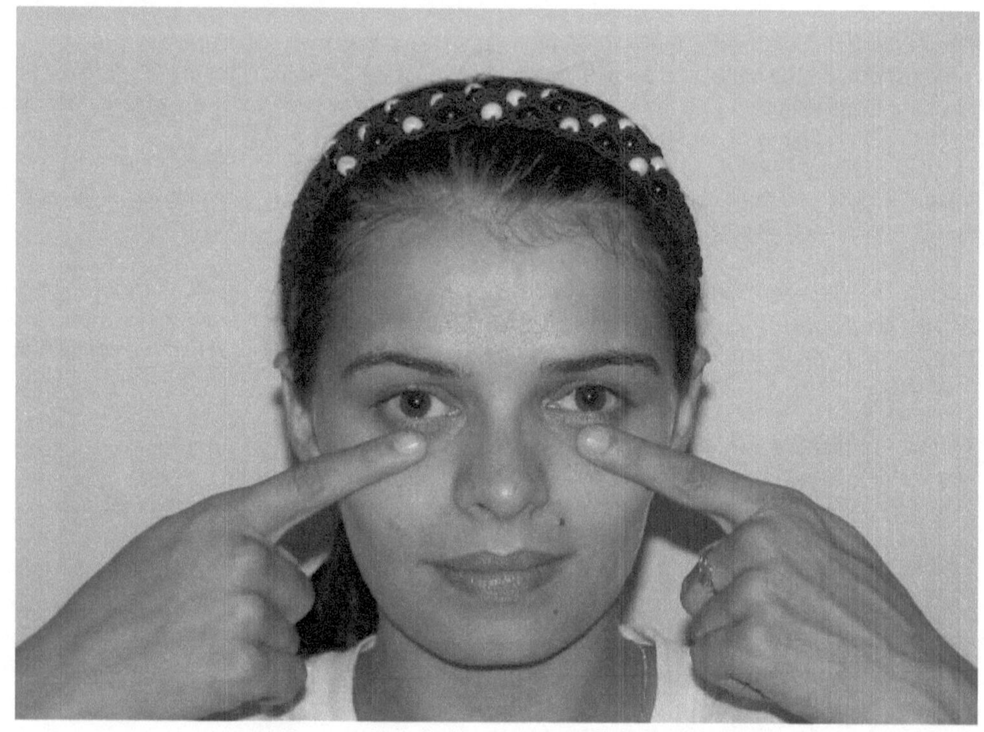

3.1.7.2. Point 7 Side View

Point 7 Side View

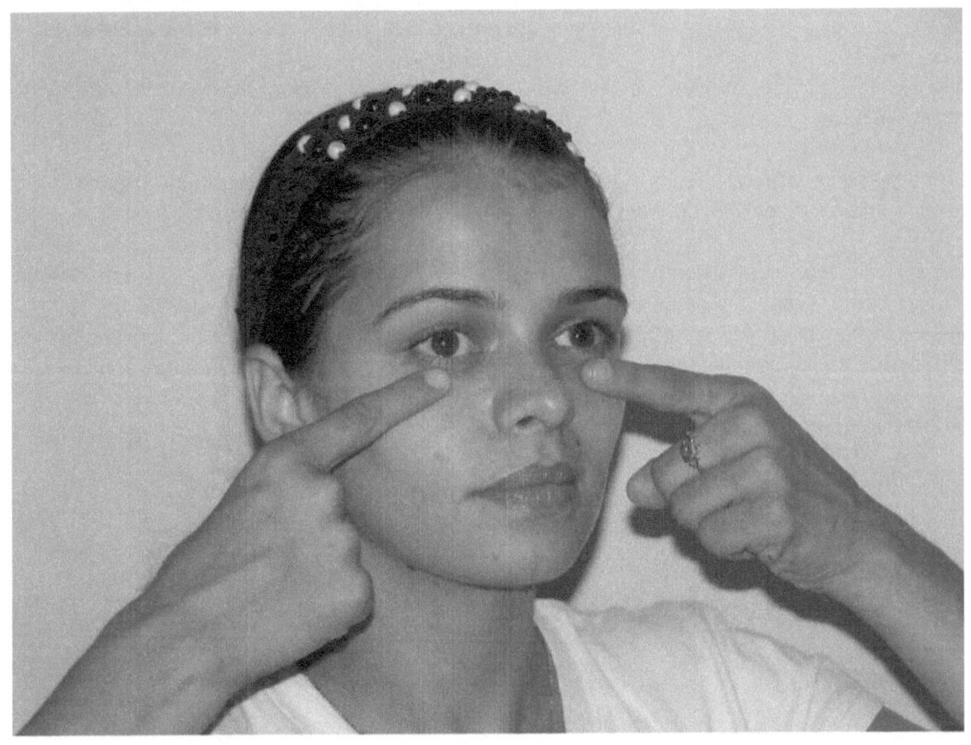

3.1.8. Facial Exercise Point 8

Location: Directly below point 7, in line with the pupils, horizontally across and in line with the flare of the nostrils. The position is in the cheek depression, just under the apex of the cheekbone.

Motion: Make small, outward circles in the cheek depression, for at least one minute, with the index fingers.

Primary Target: Chubby cheeks, hollow cheeks, smile lines and nasolabial folds, sagging face skin, jowls, sunken eye sockets, double chin, refresh skin color and glow

Benefit: This face workout enhances the large muscle of the cheeks, thereby filling and firming the sunken tissue, and will improve the natural mid-face structure. For chubby cheeks, the same facial exercise will help reduce them for a leaner face. Massaging the acupressure points here will induce blood flow, and widen the energy channels, which will improve color to the middle and lower face.

Oriental Acupressure Name: *Sibai*

Other Effects: This regimen also assists in clearing and maintaining the sinuses.

3.1.8.1. Point 8 Front View

Point 8 Front View

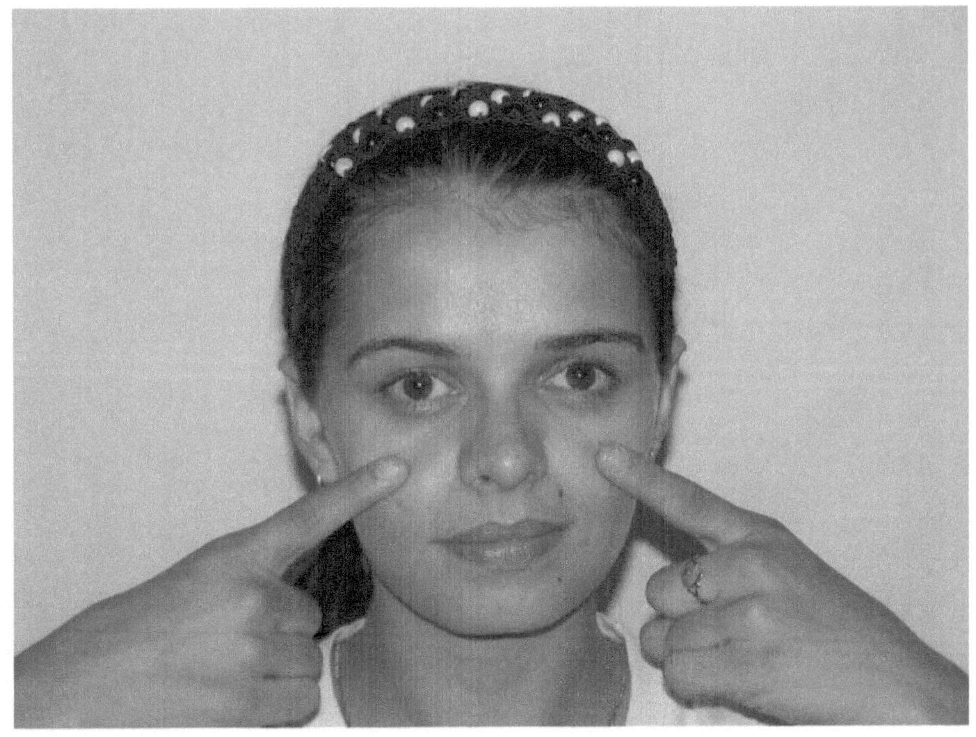

3.1.8.2. Point 8 Side View

Point 8 Side View

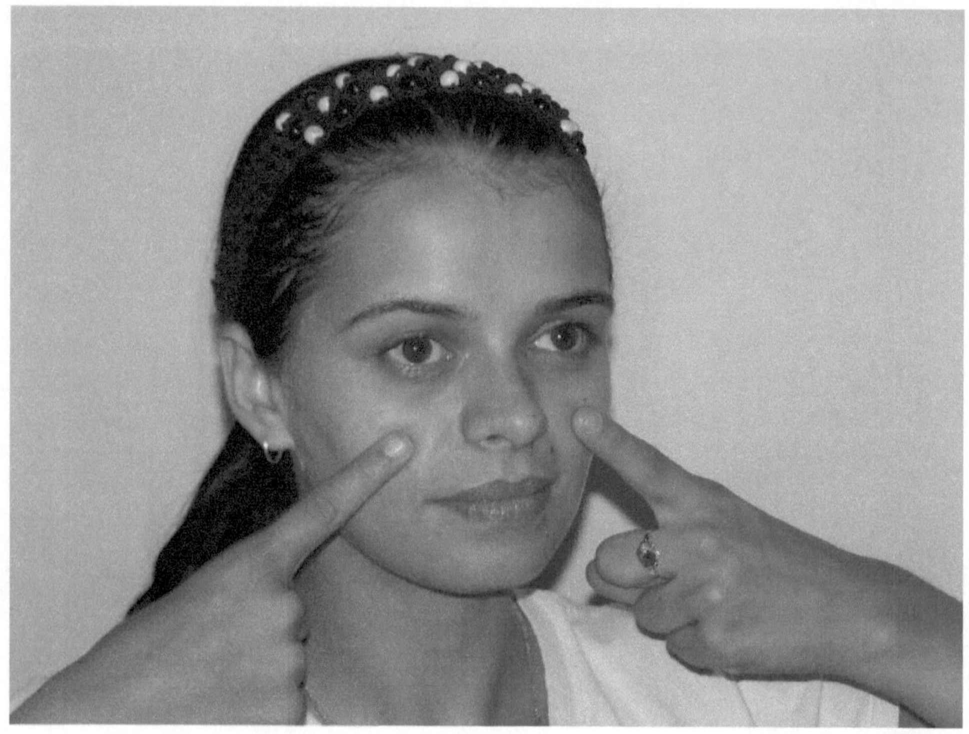

3.1.9. Facial Exercise Point 9

Location: Midway between the bottom of the nose and the top of the lip. It is in the natural cleft between the cartilage of your nose and the upper middle part of your lip, and in line with the nose bridge.

Motion: Make small, firm, clockwise circles, for at least one minute, with the index fingers.

Primary Target: Smile lines and nasolabial folds, fine lines above the lips, wrinkles around the mouth, sagging face skin

Benefit: This workout treats the vertical lines and fine wrinkles that form below the nose, and along the upper lip.

Oriental Acupressure Name: *Ren Zhong*

Other Effects: This acupressure technique is also used to alleviate fainting, dizziness, and nausea.

3.1.9.1. Point 9 Front View

Point 9 Front View

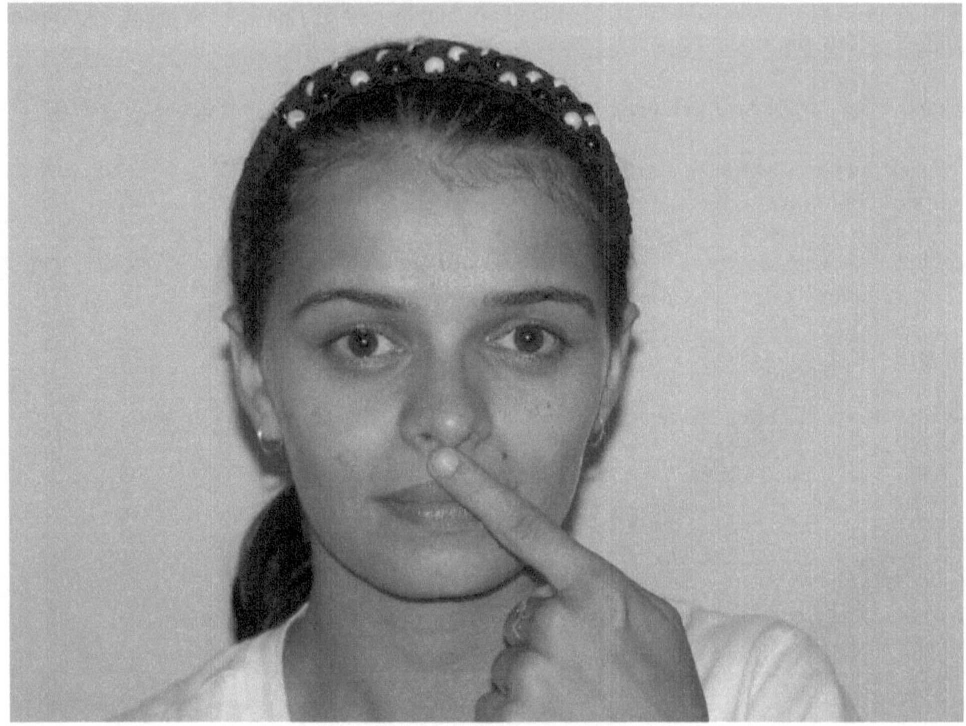

3.1.9.2. Point 9 Side View

Point 9 Side View

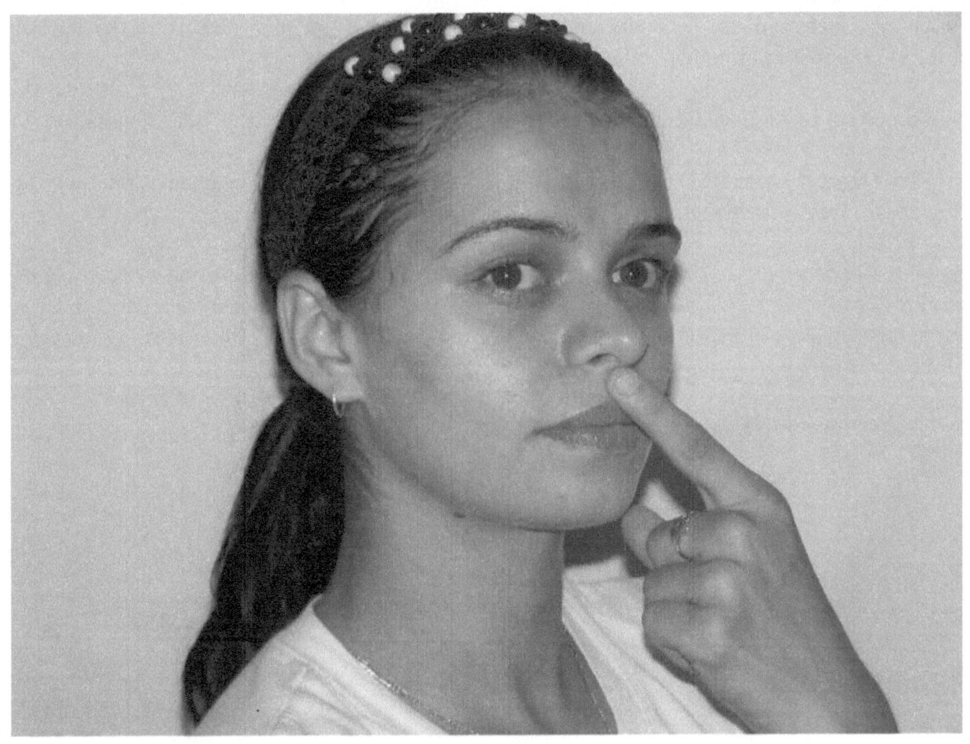

3.1.10. Facial Exercise Point 10

Location: Above the upper lip, about half an inch from the outside edges of the lips, usually on the nasal lines that manifest from the edge of the nostrils to the outer corners of the lips. These furrows are sometimes known as laughter, or smile lines.

Motion: Make small, firm outward circles, for at least one minute, with the index fingers.

Primary Target: Marionette folds and laugh lines, mouth wrinkles, hollow cheeks, fine lines above the mouth, sagging face skin, jowls, refresh skin color and glow

Benefit: This face workout minimizes the creases and lines that appear around the corners of the mouth. Sometimes these lines are very deep, and eventually become folds. This regimen will make these folds shallower, as the skin tightens over the expanded muscle with repeated massage over time.

Oriental Acupressure Name: *Dicang*

3.1.10.1. Point 10 Front View

Point 10 Front View

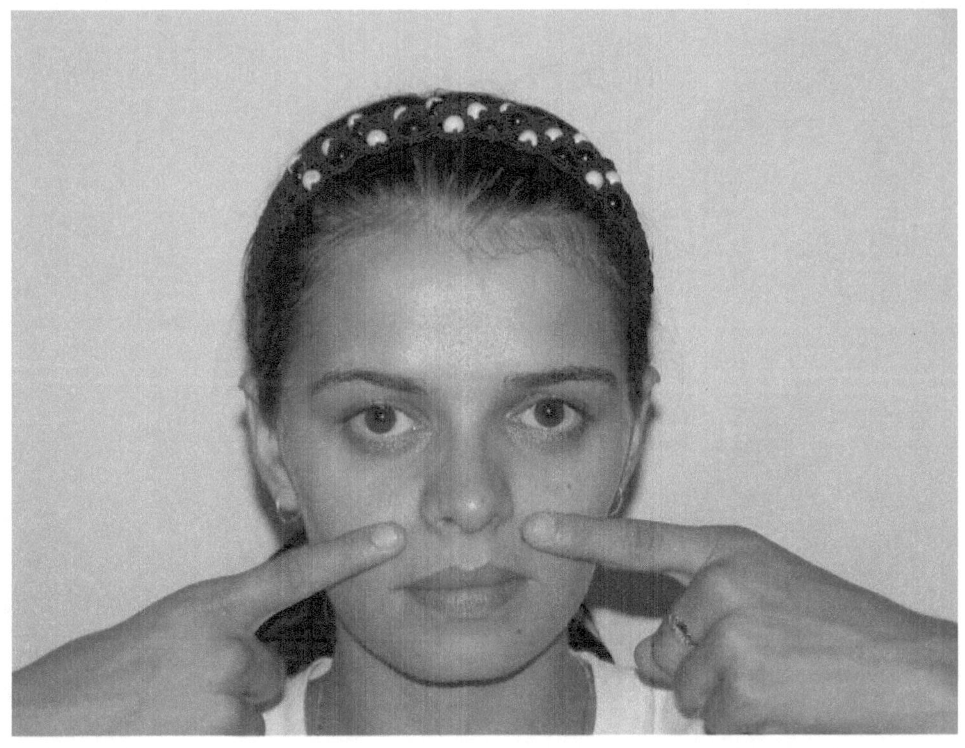

3.1.10.2. Point 10 Side View

Point 10 Side View

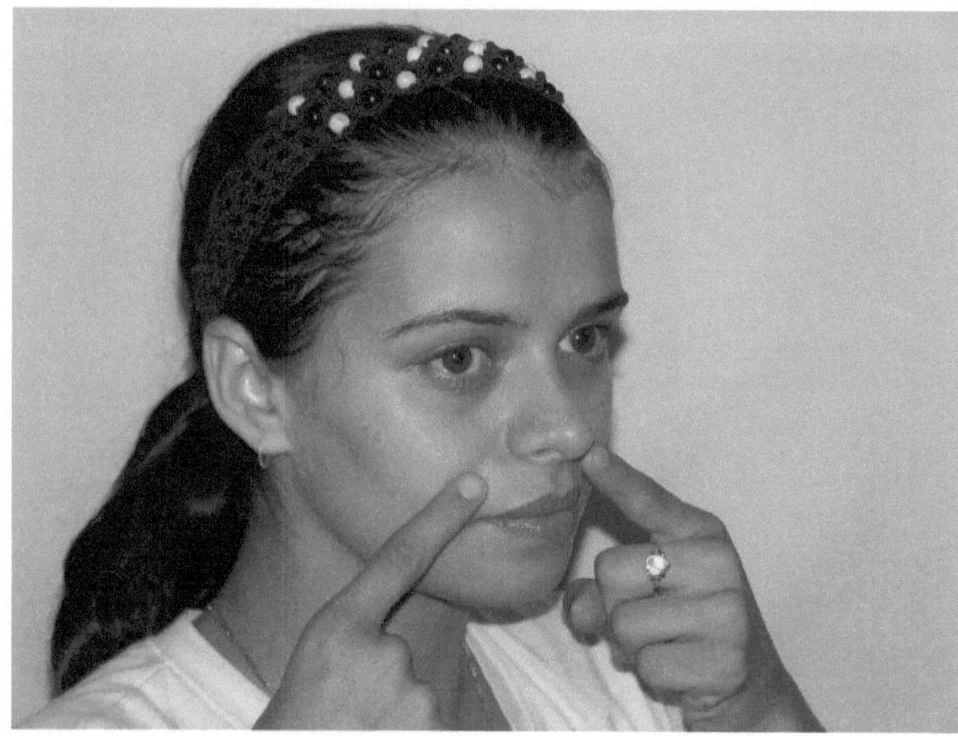

3.1.11. Facial Exercise Point 11

Location: In line with the bridge of your nose, midway between your chin and lower lip, in the natural depression that lies here.

Motion: Perform small, firm, clockwise circles, for at least one minute, with the right index finger.

Primary Target: Double chin, smile lines, fine wrinkles under and above the mouth

Benefit: This face workout minimizes chin wrinkles and reduces a double chin. It also fades lines around the mouth. It helps to energize the skin and tissue around the mouth and lower face. You will sometimes experience a tingling sensation in the lower face, when massaging this point.

Oriental Acupressure Name: *Cheng Jiang*

Other Effects: This facial exercise can have a soothing effect on lower jaw tension and headaches.

3.1.11.1. Point 11 Front View

Point 11 Front View

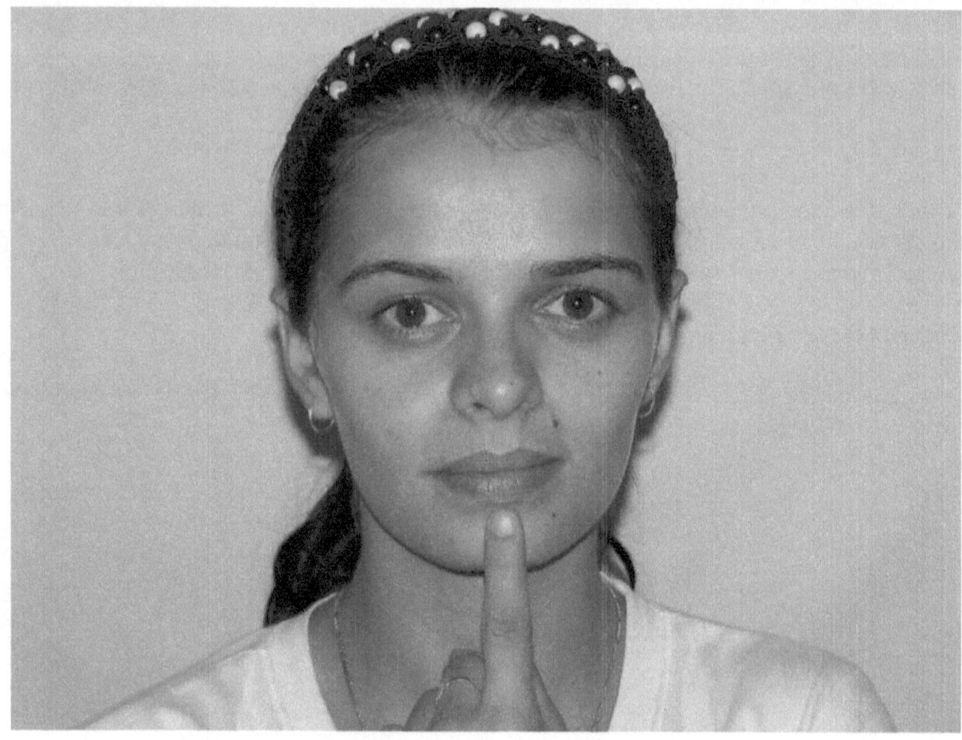

3.1.11.2. Point 11 Side View

Point 11 Side View

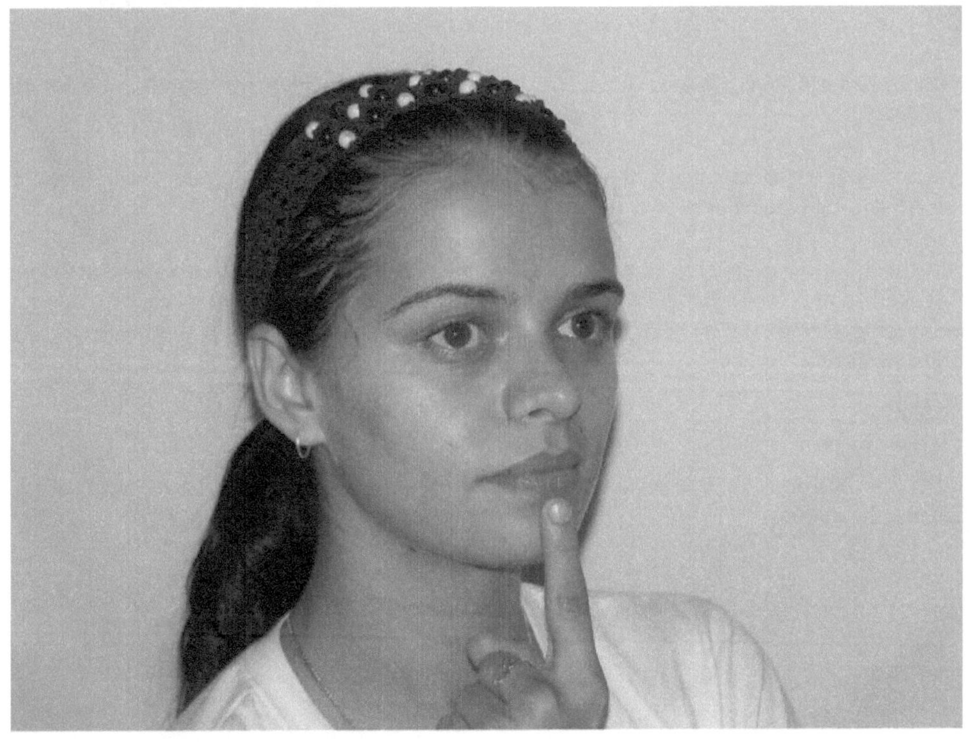

3.1.12. Facial Exercise Point 12

Location: On the big muscle at the hinge of the jaw. Allow your mouth to fall slightly open. You will find a small depression at the point of your jaw hinge.

Motion: Perform small, upward circles for at least one minute, with the forefingers, starting at the jaw hinge.

Primary Target: Hollow cheeks, chubby cheeks, sagging face skin, jowls, smile lines, double chin, refresh skin color and glow

Benefit: This facial exercise will help to lift sagging face skin and jowls, and also energize the entire face, and remedy hollow cheeks. If you have chubby cheeks, these become slimmer due to the muscles tightening on the cheek bone with repeated exercise. You might feel a tingling sensation while massaging this point.

Oriental Acupressure Name: *Chia Che*

Other Effects: This acupressure workout has a relaxing effect on lower and upper jaw tension, and can ease headaches.

3.1.12.1. Point 12 Front View

Point 12 Front View

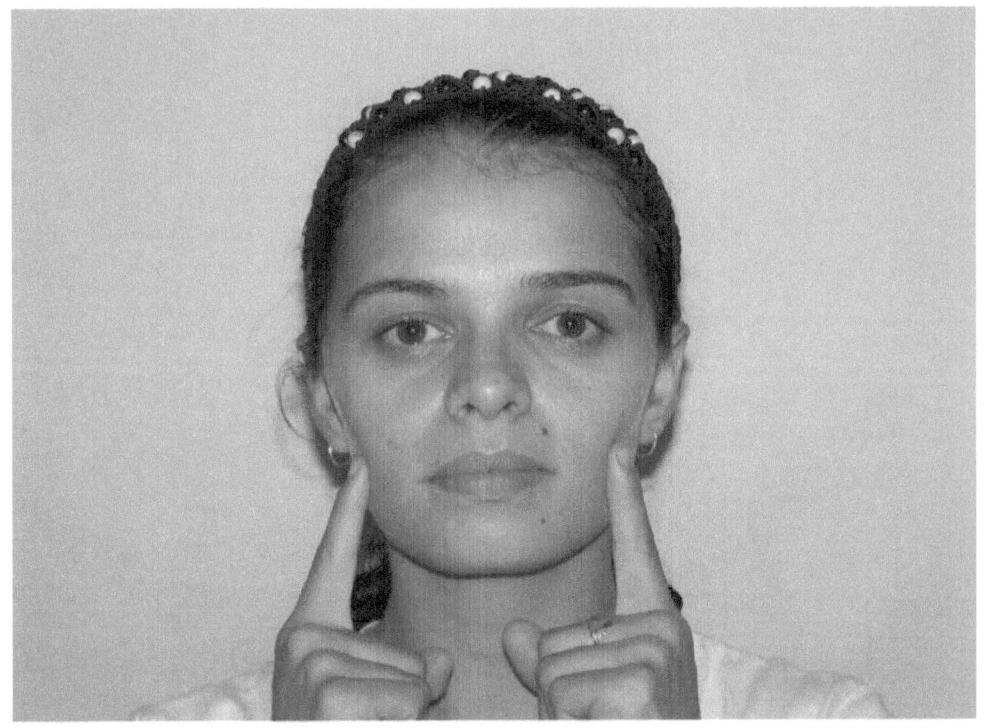

3.1.12.2. Point 12 Side View

Point 12 Side View

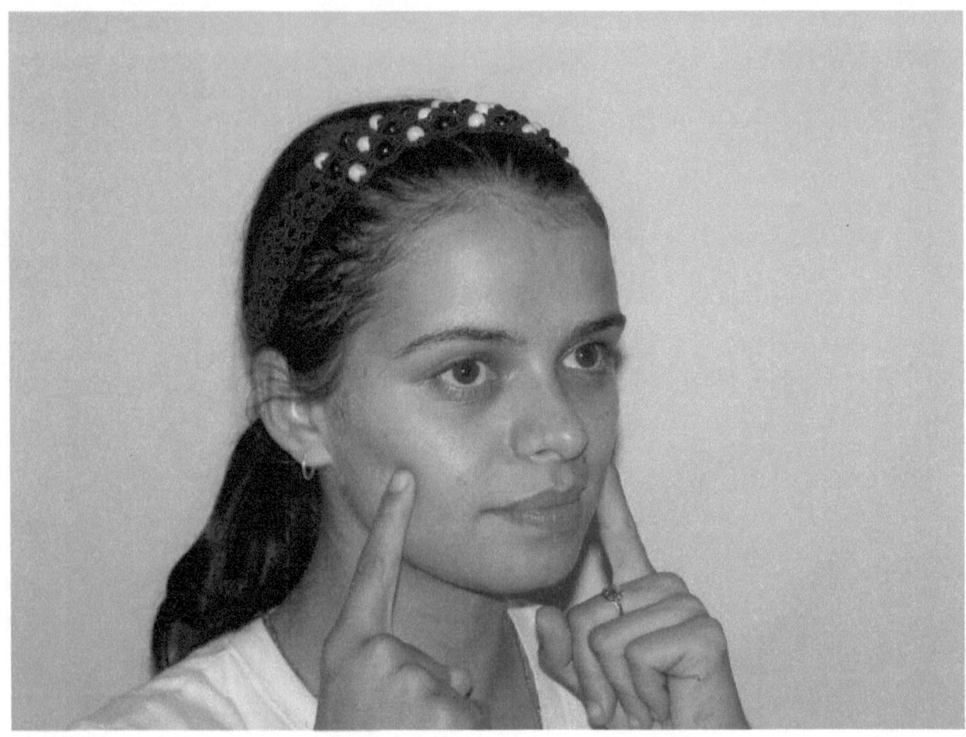

3.1.13. Facial Exercise Point 13

Location: Midway between your chin and lower lip, about half an inch below the bottom lip, and in line with the edges of the mouth.

Motion: Make small outward circles, using firm pressure with the forefingers, for at least one minute.

Primary Target: Double chin, sagging face skin, jowls, mouth wrinkles, smile lines

Benefit: This regimen minimizes lines and creases at the corners of the mouth and chin. It also firms the chin, and tightens sagging jowls and excess lower face skin.

3.1.13.1. Point 13 Front View

Point 13 Front View

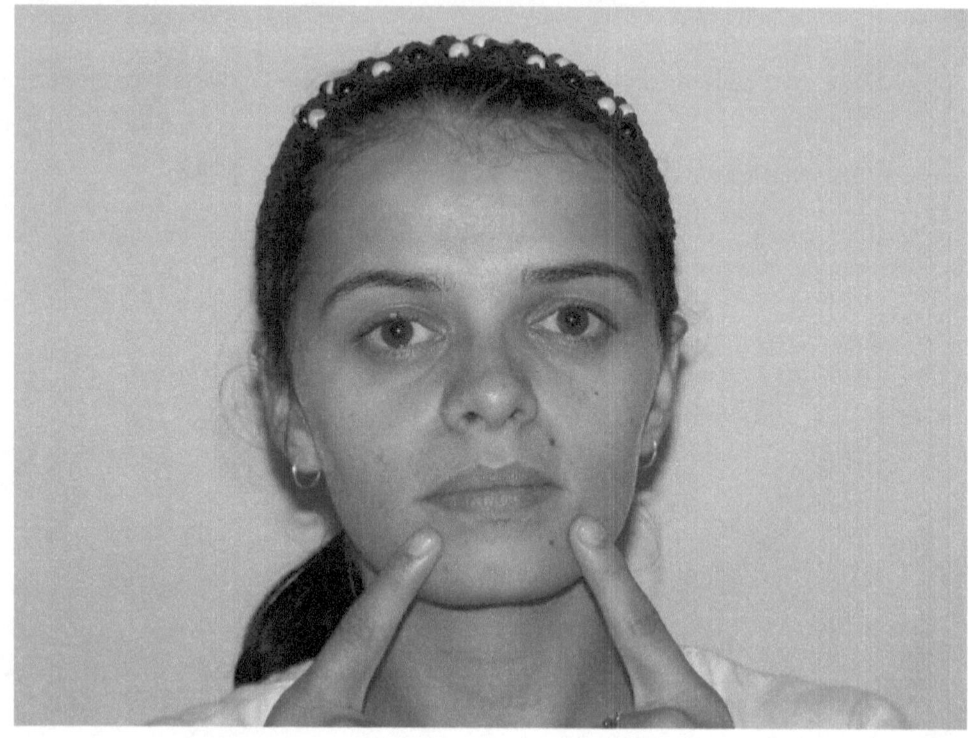

3.1.13.2. Point 13 Side View

Point 13 Side View

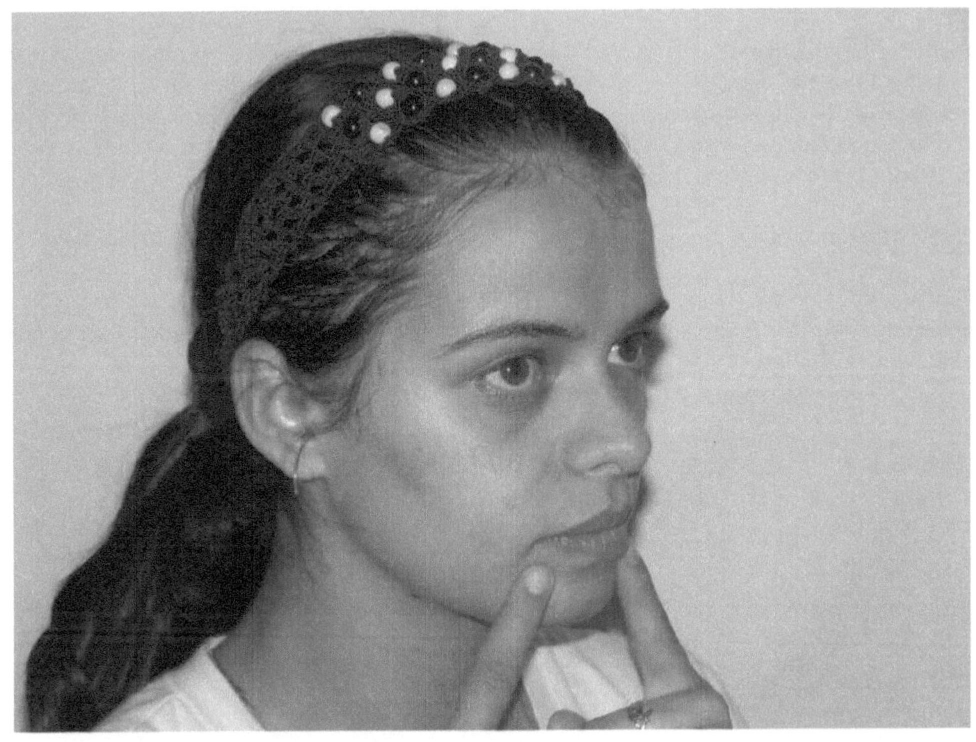

3.1.14. Chin Slap Point 14

Location: Directly below the chin, and along the entire underside of the lower jaw.

Motion: Quick rhythmic slapping. Stick your chin out when performing this regimen. Stiffen your hand, and use the back of it to conduct the slapping, while moving from ear to chin. You can employ both hands simultaneously for each side of the face, if you wish. Do not execute this regimen too hard; just enough to feel the blood flow into the bottom part of your face. Do this facial workout for one to two minutes.

Primary Target: Sagging face skin, jowls, double chin, turkey neck, refresh skin color and glow

Benefit: This rhythmic slapping technique will firm up the sagging face muscle and tissue on the underside of the jaw. It also helps to reduce double chin, and pull taut wrinkly turkey neck skin.

3.1.14.1. Point 14 Front View

Point 14 Front View

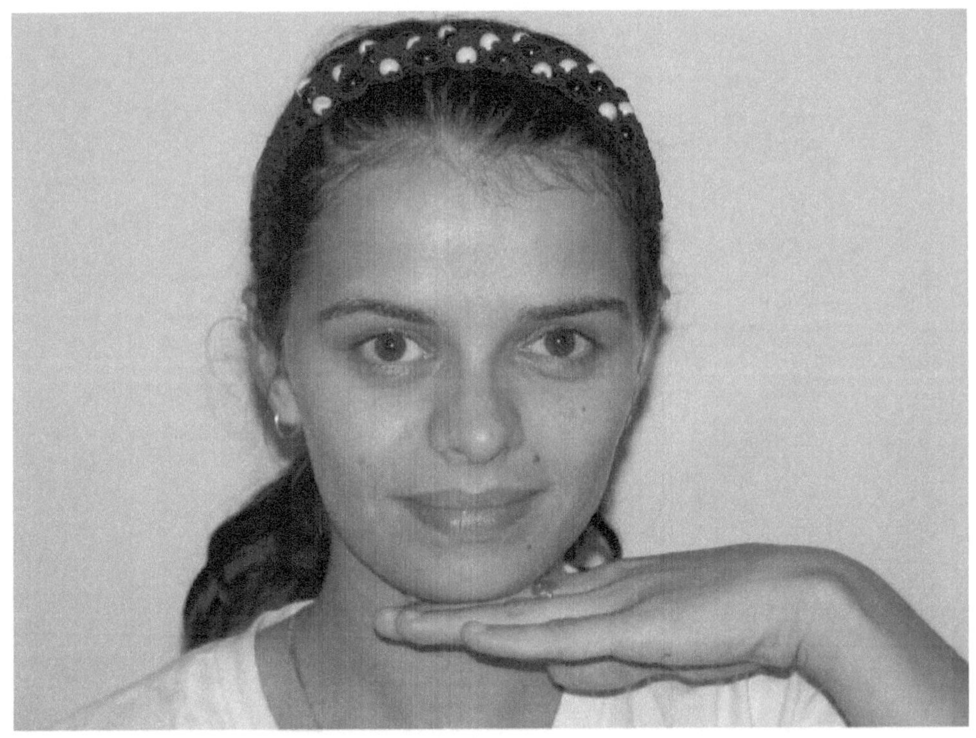

3.1.14.2. Point 14 Side View

Point 14 Side View

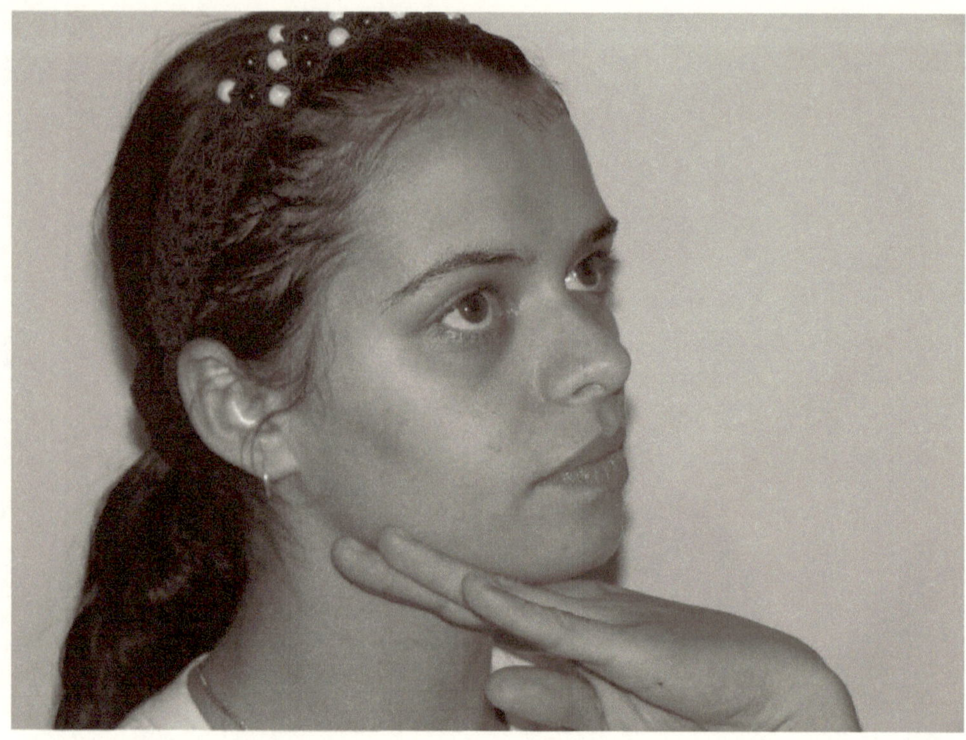

3.1.15. Facial Exercise Point 15

Location: Middle of the neck, on either side of your windpipe. Lean back slightly, and look up at the ceiling to get the right position.

Motion: Push the index fingers into the muscles on either side of the windpipe, and then move up and down with a quick, firm motion. The skin should shift with the fingers, but not be unnecessarily stretched. Do not press hard enough to restrict breathing. Practice this technique for at least one minute.

Primary Target: Turkey neck, gaunt neck, open energy points, refresh skin color and glow, improve blood flow

Benefit: This workout tightens turkey neck and smoothes out lined neck skin. It also tones local neck muscles, and combats flabby tissue and skin around the throat area.

Oriental Acupressure Name: *Ren Ying*

Other Effects: Stimulates the thyroid gland region, and generates more energy and blood flow throughout the body.

3.1.15.1. Point 15 Front View

Point 15 Front View

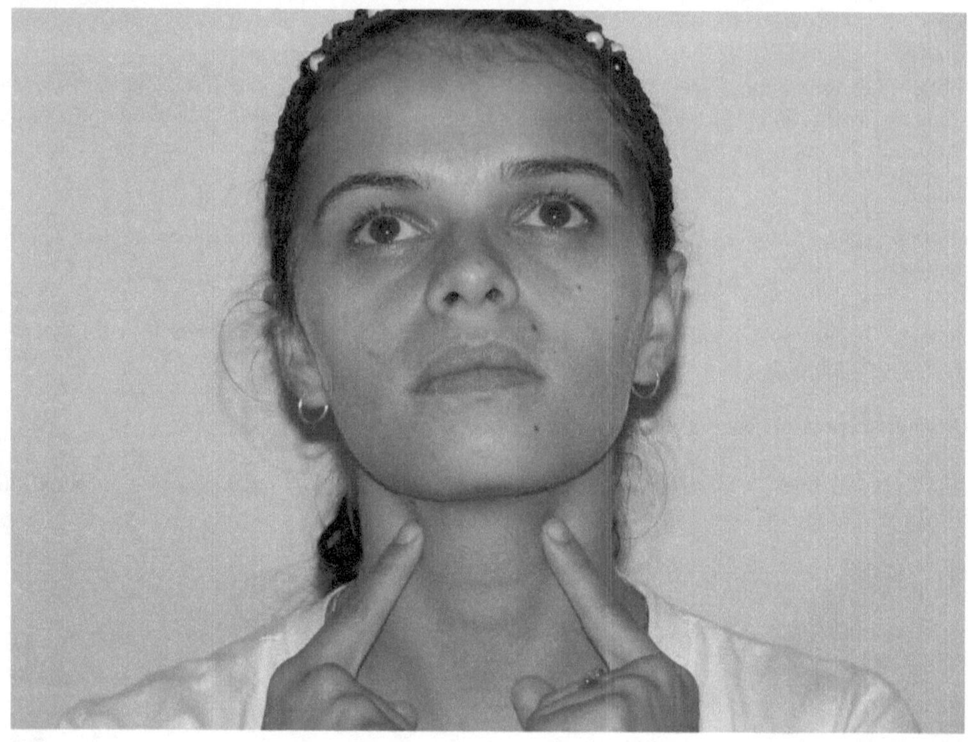

Point 15 Side View

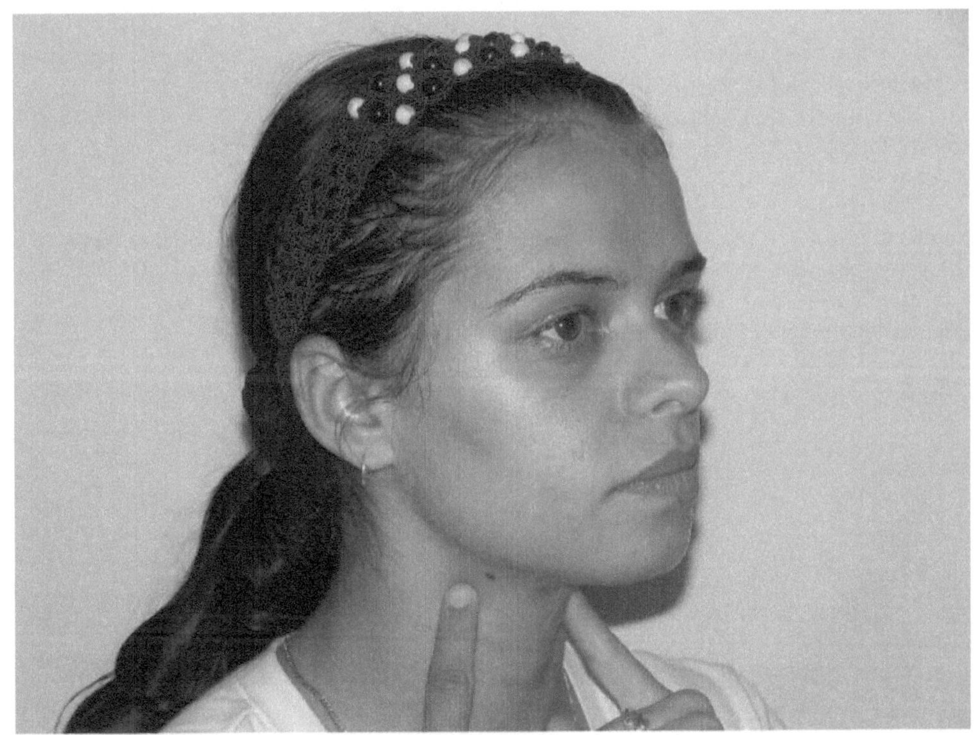

3.1.16. Facial Exercise Point 16

Location: At the base of the throat, in the notch of the diaphragm bone.

Motion: Make small tight circles on the bone with the right index finger, taking care not to restrict airflow through your windpipe. Do this regimen for at least one minute.

Primary Target: Turkey neck, gaunt neck, induce skin color and glow, open energy points, increase blood flow

Benefit: This exercise channels energy upward from the body into the neck and face region. It also reduces turkey neck, and adds color to the skin on the face and neck.

Oriental Acupressure Name: *Tian Tu*

Other Effects: This regimen is also effective in the relief of coughs and hoarseness of the throat.

3.1.16.1. Point 16 Front View

Point 16 Front View

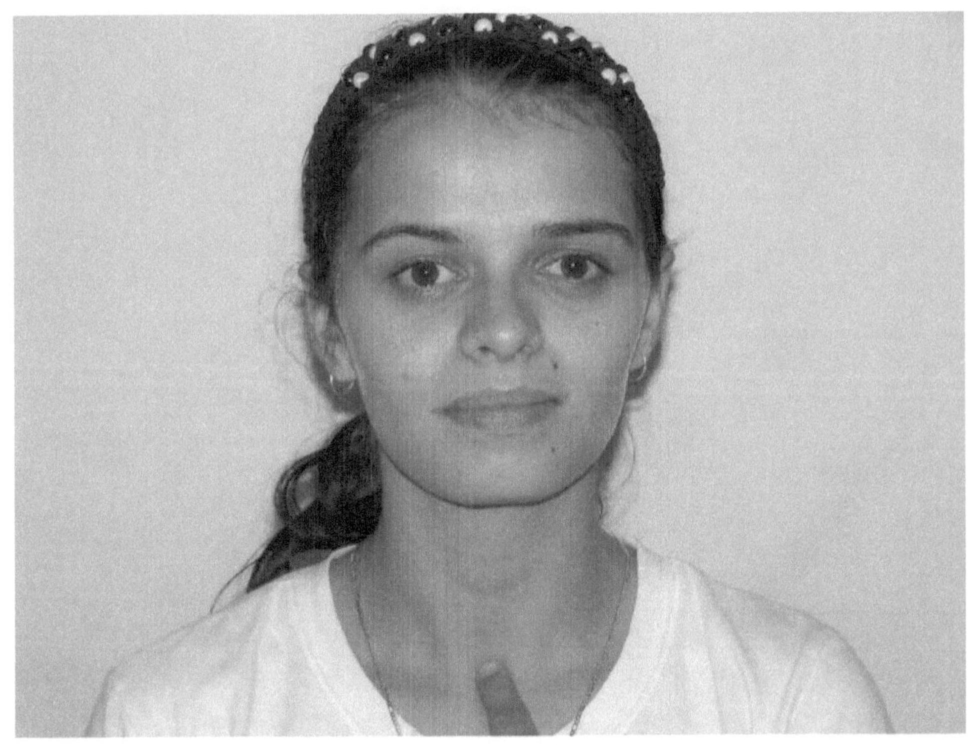

Point 16 Side View

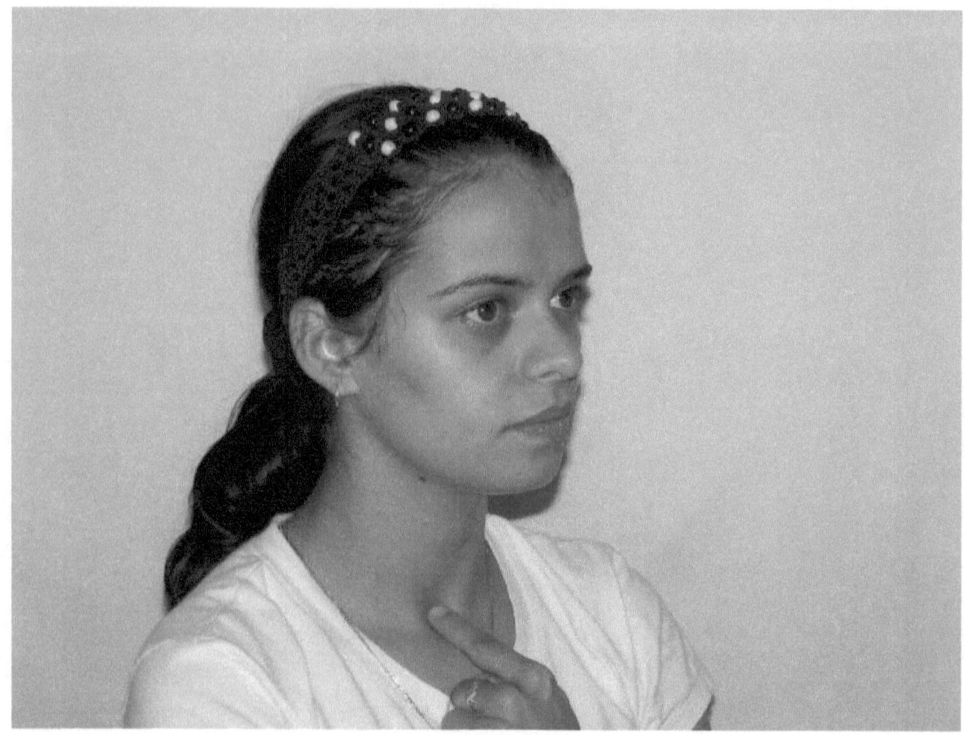

3.1.17. Acupressure Exercise Point 17

Location: On the soft web on the left hand, between the forefinger and thumb.

Motion: Massage on the web of the left hand, as deep in the groove of the hand as possible, using the tips of your thumb and forefinger of your right hand. Perform this workout for at least one minute.

Primary Target: Open the energy points, clear the meridians to the face and neck, boost the effects of all the other facial exercises

Benefit: This is one of the most important channel points - to direct energy to the neck and head region.

Oriental Acupressure Name: *Ho Ku*

Other Effects: This point is commonly used to combat headaches and toothache, and can also boost digestion.

3.1.17.1. Point 17 Front View

Point 17 Front View

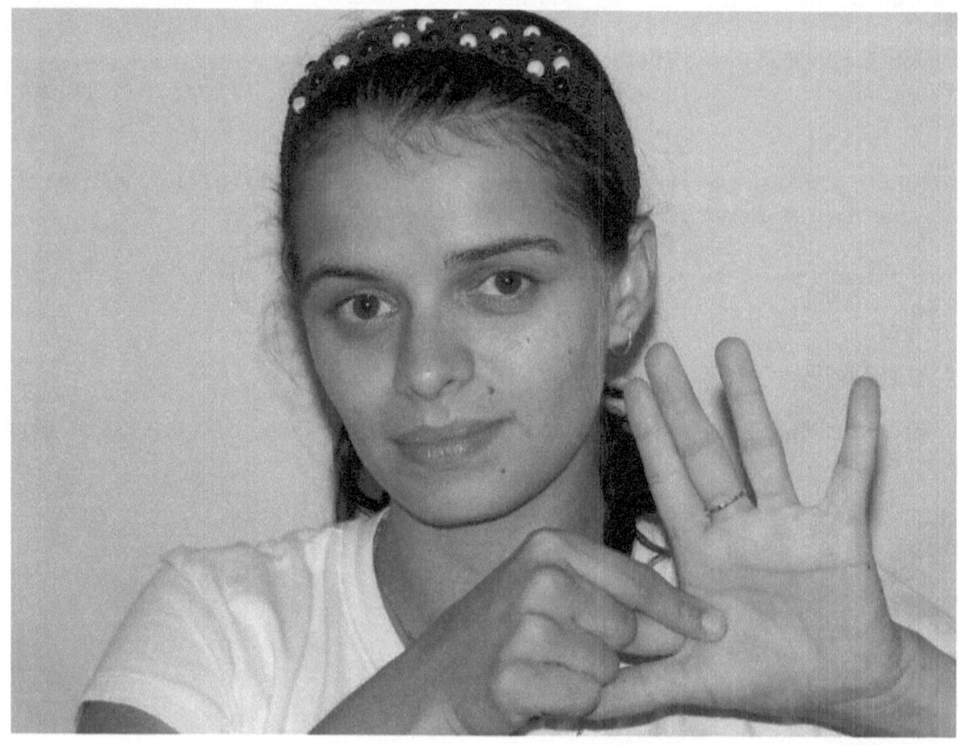

3.1.18. Acupressure Exercise Point 18

Location: On the soft web on the right hand, between the forefinger and thumb.

Motion: Massage on the web of the right hand, as deep in the groove of the hand as possible, using the tips of your thumb and forefinger of your left hand. Perform this workout for at least one minute.

Primary Target: Open the energy points, clear the meridians to the face and neck, boost the effects of all the other facial exercises.

Benefit: This is one of the most important channel points of the entire body - to direct energy to the neck and head region.

Oriental Acupressure Name: *Ho Ku*

Other Effects: This point is commonly used to combat headaches and toothache, and can also boost digestion.

3.1.18.1. Point 18 Front View

Point 18 Front View

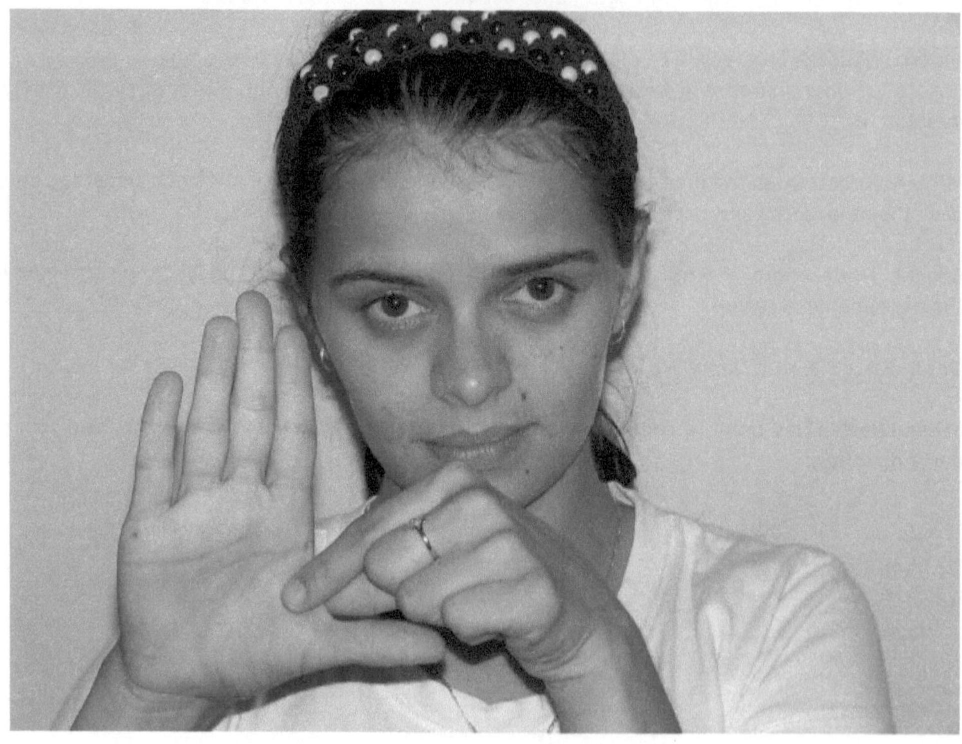

3.1.19. Acupressure Point 19

Location: At the base of the crease of the left elbow. Place the left hand on the right shoulder. Push in the right thumb into the groove at the base of the crease of the left arm. You will discover a small notch against the bone. It is in this notch that you will locate the point.

Motion: With your right thumb, massage deep into this notch, using a small, circular motion for at least one minute.

Primary Target: Open the energy points, clear the meridians to the face and neck, boost the effects of all the other facial exercises.

Benefit: This workout channels energy and increases blood flow to the neck, face, and entire head.

Oriental Acupressure Name: *Chu Chih*

Other Effects: This regimen treats the skin of the entire body.

3.1.19.1. Point 19 Front View

Point 19 Front View

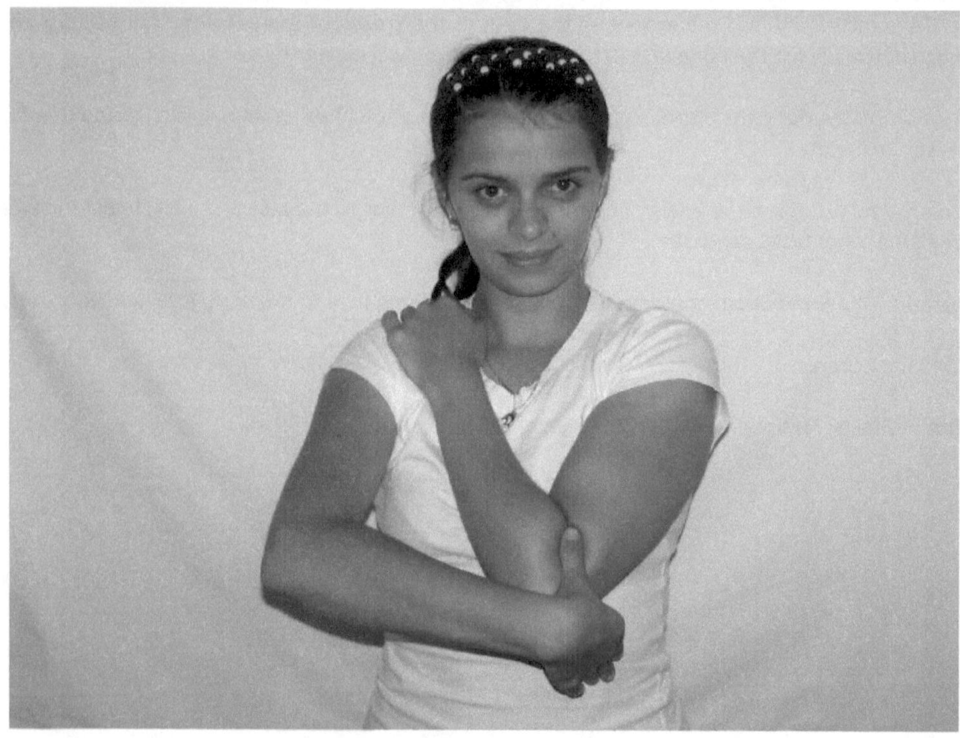

3.1.20. Acupressure Point 20

Location: At the base of the crease of the right elbow. Place the right hand on the left shoulder. Push in the left thumb into the groove at the base of the crease of the right arm. You will discover a small notch against the bone. It is in this notch that you will locate the point.

Motion: With your left thumb, massage deep into this notch, using a small, circular motion for at least one minute.

Primary Target: Open the energy points and meridians to the face and neck, boost the effects of all the other facial exercises.

Benefit: This workout channels energy and increases blood flow to the neck, face, and entire head.

Oriental Acupressure Name: *Chu Chih*

Other Effects: This regimen treats the skin of the entire body.

3.1.20.1. Point 20 Front View

Point 20 Front View

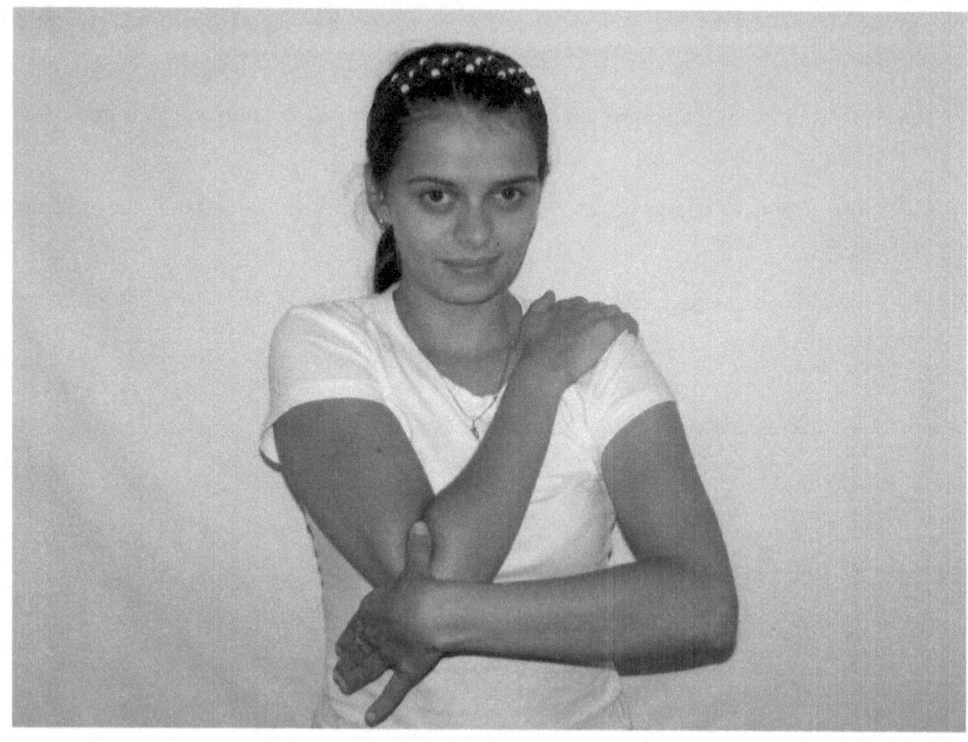

3.2. Face And Neck Exercises For Specific Problem Areas

Each person is unique, and has certain areas on their face that they could feel need attention. I have compiled the best face workouts to use, for problem areas that you might experience on your face and neck:

Forehead Lines: Perform regimens for points 1 to 20 for one minute each, to open the energy points and increase blood flow. Then redo points 1, 2, 3 for one to four minutes on each point. You can always do these problem areas again later in the day or evening, if you have time.

Crow's Feet: Perform regimens for points 1 to 20 for one minute each, to open the energy points and increase blood flow. Then redo points 5, 6, 7 for one to four minutes on each point. You can always do these problem areas again later in the day or evening, if you have time.

Dark Eye Circles: Perform regimens for points 1 to 20 for one minute each, to open the energy points and increase blood flow. Then redo points 4, 5, 6, 7 for one to four minutes on each point. You can always do these problem areas again later in the day or evening, if you have time. Try to get more sleep nightly. Take a daily oral Vitamin K supplement, as recommended on the bottle (RDA – Recommended Daily Allowance). Drink at least 8 glasses of water or organic fruit juice daily, as dark circles can be a symptom of kidney complications.

Eye Bags: Perform regimens for points 1 to 20 for one minute each, to open the energy points and increase blood flow. Then redo points 4, 5, 6, 7 for one to four minutes on each point. You can always do these problem areas again later in the day or evening, if you have time.

Hollow And Sunken Eyes: Perform regimens for points 1 to 20 for one minute each, to open the energy points and increase blood flow. Then redo points 6, 7, 8 for one to four minutes on each point. You can always do these problem areas again later in the day or evening, if you have time.

Under Eye Wrinkles: Perform regimens for points 1 to 20 for one minute each, to open the energy points and increase blood flow. Then redo points 4, 5, 6, 7 for one to four minutes on each point. You can always do these problem areas again later in the day or evening, if you have time.

Chubby And Sagging Cheeks: Perform regimens for points 1 to 20 for one minute each, to open the energy points and increase blood flow. Then redo points 7, 8, 12 for one to four minutes on each point. You can always do these problem areas again later in the day or evening, if you have time.

Gaunt And Hollow Cheeks: Perform regimens for points 1 to 20 for one minute each, to open the energy points and increase blood flow. Then redo points 8, 10, 12 for one to four minutes on each point. You can always do these problem areas again later in the day or evening, if you have time.

Smile Lines And Nasolabial Folds: Perform regimens for points 1 to 20 for one minute each, to open the energy points and increase blood flow. Then redo points 8, 9, 10, 11, 12 for one to four minutes on each point. You can always do these problem areas again later in the day or evening, if you have time.

Fine Lines Above The Lips: Perform regimens for points 1 to 20 for one minute each, to open the energy points and increase blood flow. Then redo points 9, 10, 11 for one to four minutes on each point. You can always do these problem areas again later in the day or evening, if you have time.

Sagging Face Skin And Jowls: Perform regimens for points 1 to 20 for one minute each, to open the energy points and increase blood flow. Then redo points 8, 10, 12, 14 for one to four minutes on each point. You can always do these problem areas again later in the day or evening, if you have time.

Double Chin: Perform regimens for points 1 to 20 for one minute each, to open the energy points and increase blood flow. Then redo points 8, 11, 12, 13, 14 for one to four minutes on each point. You can always do these problem areas again later in the day or evening, if you have time.

Turkey Neck And Lined Neck: Perform regimens for points 1 to 20 for one minute each, to open the energy points and increase blood flow. Then redo points 14, 15, 16 for one to four minutes on each point. You can always do these problem areas again later in the day or evening, if you have time.

Gaunt And Thin Neck: Perform regimens for points 1 to 20 for one minute each, to open the energy points and increase blood flow. Then redo points 15, 16 for one to four minutes on each point. You can always do these problem areas again later in the day or evening, if you have time.

Pale And Colorless Skin: Perform regimens for points 1 to 20 for one minute each, to open the energy points and increase blood flow. Then redo points 2, 7, 8, 10, 12, 14, 15 for one to four minutes on each point. You can always do these problem areas again later in the day or evening, if you have time. Take daily oral Vitamin A, C, E supplements as directed on the bottles (RDA – Recommended Daily Allowance)

As regards to any substance or Vitamin intake mentioned in this book, please do not ingest anything that we might recommend that is contrary to a medical expert's advice. If in doubt, please consult you medical practitioner.

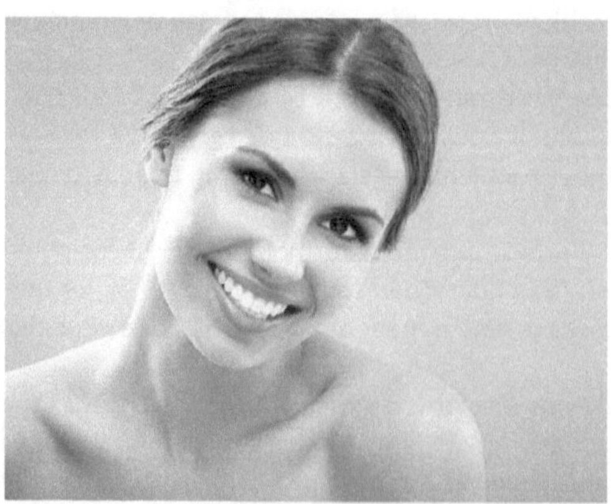

3.3. Facial Exercises – A Shortened Version For Those Pressed For Time

Many people have asked me for a shortened version of the acupressure face toning program. I always advise that men and women should rigorously practice all 20 points, to enjoy the full benefits of wrinkle elimination and the tightening of saggy skin. However, I do realize this is a modern "pressure cooker" society we live in, and that some folks just do not get time to sit down for at least 20 minutes a day, for the first month of commencing this system.

I have thus selected the 10 MOST IMPORTANT FACE EXERCISE POINTS to do, as a shortened version of the Facial Regeneration Exercises program: Please ensure that you perform at least these 10 facial workouts:

Points 2, 3, 6, 7, 8, 10, 12, 13, 14, 15 for one minute each. Problem areas such as those depicted under the heading "Face And Neck Exercises For Specific Problem Areas" should also be addressed.

If you have spare time available in the week, you can always resort to the full 20 point version of the program.

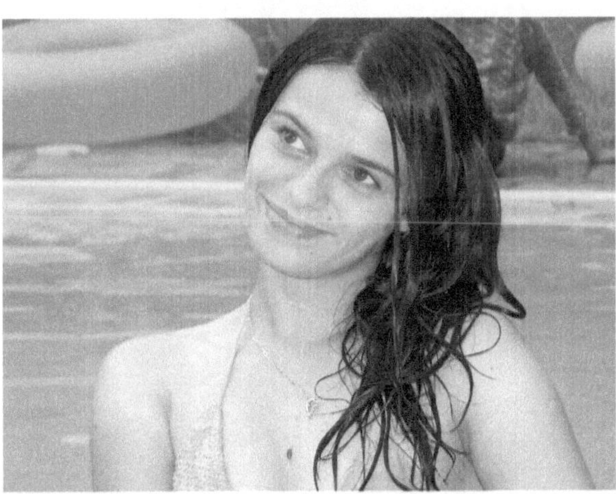

4. SECTION 4
4.1. How To Boost Your Face Exercise Efforts For Quicker Results

Tip 1: Remove all makeup and base before commencing your facial exercise regimens. This is because it is best to allow your skin to breathe while you tone.

Tip 2: Apply moisturizer to the face and neck. Do not use thick moisturizers that have the tendency to clog up the skin pores. I personally use Nivea Rich Nourishing Body Moisturizer for dry skin on my face, even though it has the words "Body" on the plastic bottle. You can Google it to see whether it is available in your country. Nivea is a rich cream that nourishes skin cells and is ideal for face exercises. Do not apply too much lotion; just enough to get the skin soft and supple to the touch.

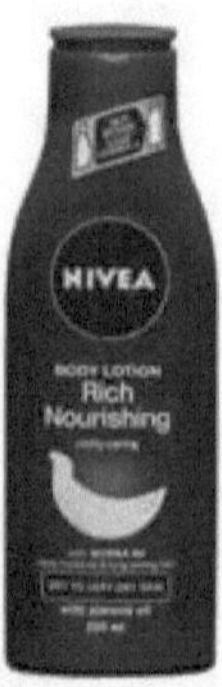

Tip 3: Try to relax and breathe steadily, as you perform the routines. This will oxygenate the blood, and help open the energy meridians - so you can get the full benefit of the face workouts.

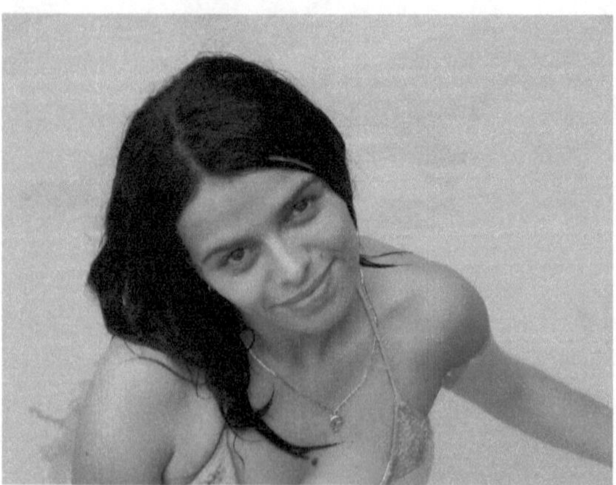

4.2. What Not To Do With Face Exercises

1. PLEASE DO NOT use another facial exercise, or face yoga system, while you are applying the Facial Regeneration Exercises regimens. This is because many of these programs employ a system of isometrics. The Facial Regeneration Exercises program applies facial toning on nodal acupressure points, for optimum results. Using facial isometrics, together with toning, can be counter-productive - because you will be overdoing things, and stressing the facial and neck tissue. Apply the techniques in this program only, OR somebody else's only, BUT NOT BOTH PROGRAMS AT THE SAME TIME.

2. Do not overdo the facial exercises. It is human nature to go overboard when people witness the wrinkles fading, and the skin tightening. Overdoing these face regimens can be a bad thing. Much like exercising in the gym, "Train, but do not strain" is an adage that bodybuilders frequently use. Often, it is beneficial to give it a rest for a day or two, to allow the muscles to settle before resuming facial exercises. Usually your body will tell you that you are overdoing things e.g. you do not see improvements anymore, parts of your face or neck are tender to the touch, or you experience slight bruising. Rather stop for a period, and then continue. You will definitely benefit from doing this!

3. Do not push, push, push for results! Stressing and running to the mirror every 5 minutes to see if your wrinkles are fading is stressful, and counter-productive. Why? Because you must be in a relaxed state to boost the age-regression benefits you strive for. You will enjoy better results if you are at ease in your head. Acupressure facial toning is based on relaxation and harmony between your mind and body, because this keeps the energy channels open. Blood and energy flow is maximized when you are at peace with yourself, which translates to better and faster results with facial exercises.

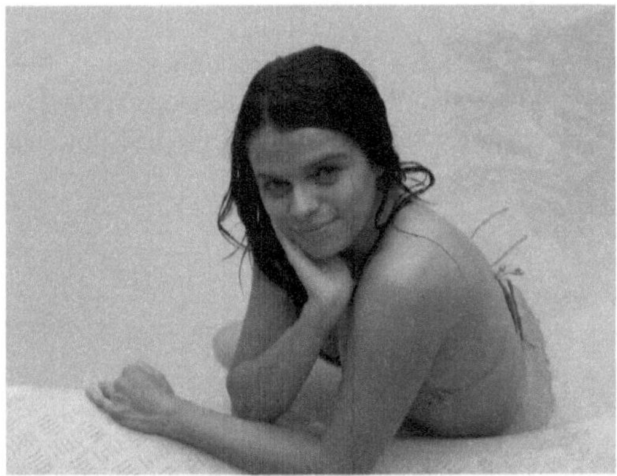

4.3. Troubleshooting Any Problems You Might Experience

There might be temporary negative effects, after starting these regimens. They are 99% of the time short-lived, because your body will adjust to the face workouts. Here are some that men and women might experience:

1. *Stuffy nose, or blocked sinuses for the first few days*: This is perfectly normal. After a few days, this should recede, as your sinuses and face tissue get accustomed to the routines.

2. *Stiffness and muscle sensitivity in the face when smiling or making facial expressions*: Again, this is normal. However, if it is uncomfortable, give the face and neck workouts a rest for a day or two. Or, avoid these sensitive areas, until the soreness has diminished. You might also be pressing too hard with your fingers into the muscles and tissue. It is advisable to ease up on the pressure when you manipulate the acupressure points.

3. *Bruising in the first days*: Some people are more prone to bruising than others. This could be due to a lack of Vitamins E and C, or could be a result of other factors. Always listen to what your body is telling you. Bruising can be an indication of massaging too hard, or overdoing it. Stop immediately in that face or neck zone. Then, resume tentatively after a few days, once the discoloration has faded. When you restart the face workouts, be gentler and more mindful of the face exercise routines.

4. *Stiff neck and shoulders*: Try to relax when performing the face exercise regimens. Your posture could be incorrect when performing them. You might not even notice this until you feel the stiffness the next day. Try to sit in a comfortable chair or sofa, lean back and relax your shoulders. Breathe deeply in and out, until you feel at ease and comfortable. If necessary, lean your head back on a head rest, and then perform the workouts.

5. *Acne breakout*: In rare cases, some people experience acne. These breakouts are usually not severe, and are a positive sign that toxins are being expelled from the face and neck, as the pores and energy channels start to open. This problem should subside after 2 to 3 weeks.

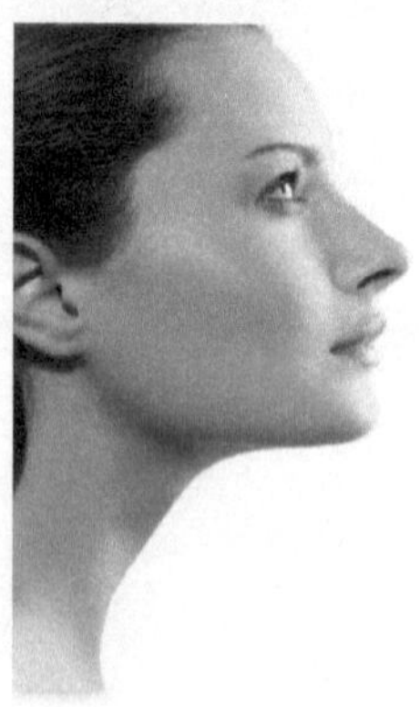

4.4. Frequently Asked Questions

Q: Does massaging the 20 acupressure points really work?
A: Yes. The principle is that it stimulates blood flow to the underlying tissue, and the skin. In fact, it is beneficial for the entire body. The principle of face toning with the fingers has been used successfully for over 3000 years.

Q: How fast will I see results?
A: Possibly the same day. After a week of basic daily massaging, for approximately one minute on each point (20 minutes in total), you and others should notice a softening of wrinkles and facial lines. You should also see renewed color in your face.

Q: How often must I apply the 20 point face massage program?
A: I recommend daily for the first 30 days, 2 to 3 times a week thereafter for maintenance. If you wish to tackle the problem areas on your face, then you can always repeat the workouts to remedy that problem, after doing the basic 20 points.

Q: What about treating problematic areas on my face such as double chin, hollow cheeks, and deep smile lines?
A: Each person's face is different. Conduct the full 20 point face exercise set, and then redo the problem areas on your face, as explained under the "Face And Neck Exercises For Specific Problem Areas".

Q: How am I going to find the time to do this?
A: It must become a habit for you - a way of life. Think about it this way: You find the time to shower, brush your teeth, dress, and eat every day, so why not spend some time performing simple face workouts to look younger and feel more confident?

Q: Are the effects permanent?
A: Yes, as long as you maintain your toning efforts every week. Much like exercise, you need to do the routines regularly to maintain the benefits, keep the skin firm and glowing, and to eradicate wrinkles.

Q: If I halt the face exercises, will my face revert to what it was before I started your program?
A: Everybody is different, but generally over a few months of not doing the acupressure facial exercises, your face will start to show signs of aging again. It is the same as giving up on exercising your body in the gym. Things resort to their previous state with lack of exercise. So, please do not stop! If you leave it for a few weeks due to things going on in your life, so be it. The sooner you kick-start the program again, the better. It is important to maintain your non-surgical facelift efforts.

Q: Will I get the best results after the first 30 days?
A: Generally, yes. Again, it depends on the individual. Age, skin type, health of the person, frequency of doing the face regimens are all factors that determine how fast and how radical the results are. Be patient. Remember, it has taken a lifetime for you to get those wrinkles and that

sagging skin. Once you feel that you have obtained the desired effect, start decreasing the regimens to a maintenance schedule of 2 to 3 times a week, or more if you wish. But remember, do not overdo things. Resting your face and neck muscles for a day, or two, or three is a good thing, because your muscles can set and get ready for further progress, with Facial Regeneration Exercises.

Q: Must I follow the same facial workout sequence from my forehead downwards, as shown in this program?
A: Yes, preferably. This is because the natural energy flow of the body is from top to bottom. You might not derive the same benefits if you massage the points in a random fashion.

Q: Does your program help eliminate sun damage and liver spots?
A: No, but it can fade them to some degree. If you start the program earlier in life, it is likely that it will minimize the opportunity of them growing on your face and neck in the first place.

Q: Can facial exercises make people look years younger in their latter years?
A: Definitely. The sooner one starts, the better. You might have to perform the workouts in the program more often, if you are further in your years, but the end result will be well worth it. A 74 year old gentleman friend I personally know tried the program, and he looked absolutely transformed after 30 days. A lot of color and thickness to his once paper thin skin was restored significantly.

Q: Can the program be practiced by men?
A: Men, women, teens – all will benefit, young and old. The pressure points are always in the same location.

Q: Will the face exercise routines lessen acne scars?
A: To some extent the system will work. As the tissue expands with exercise, scar hollows will fill out. But, keep in mind that scars are scars, and you might need other treatments, such as topical applications of tissue oil - which works wonders on healed scars.

Q: How easy is it to locate the acupressure points on which to perform the face exercises?
A: Use the pictures in this book to guide you. After a while, you will literally be able to find them with your eyes closed! I often perform the routines in front of the television, when I'm in a relaxed state.

Q: I am struggling to find the acupressure points to apply the massage techniques. What do I do now?
A: Each point shown in the pictures has a tiny depression in the underlying tissue, or on the bone of the skull, abdomen, hands, and arms. This depression is where acupuncturists place their needles to remedy certain health problems. If you cannot find the exact spot, use the pictures in the program to find the APPROXIMATE AREA of the nodal point. The closer you are, the more effective the program. Do not worry if you are unable to locate the exact acupressure spot.

Q: Must I always massage the points in front of a mirror?

A: Yes, in the beginning. It is better to conduct your face exercises in front of a mirror, with the aid of the Facial Regeneration Exercises program in front of you. This is to ensure that you have got the location of the acupressure points correct. Many people load the book onto their iPad, or Kindle, or mobile device for convenience. After a while, you will be able to perform the toning in front of the television, at the bus stop, or even on the toilet! Any opportunity you can muster is advisable, if you live a pressured lifestyle.

Q: How early in life should I start the Facial Regeneration Exercises program?
A: The earlier the better. In an ideal world, you should commence in your late teens, but alas we usually only start facial exercises when we see symptoms of aging ravaging our faces! The ancient Chinese taught us that prevention is better than cure. However, it is never too late to start!

Q: If I have not practiced the program for a long while, how may I restart?
A: Begin as if you have never applied face workouts. Go back to basics. Perform the routines daily for the first 30 days, and then go into the maintenance procedure of 2 to 3 times a week. You will observe that even before the first 30 days have elapsed, that your face will revert to a more youthful appearance a lot quicker than when you started the first time. This is because the tissue and underlying muscles have already been primed - with your prior face exercise efforts.

Q: If I have undergone cosmetic surgery in the past, will your program help me to look younger?
A: Yes, but it may take a bit longer to see an improvement. This is because the scarring and incisions from the medical procedure might hamper energy and blood flow to your face, neck, and head.

Q: I have just had Botox and fillers injected into my face. Should I still use your face exercise program?
A: I strongly advise that you do not apply the techniques described here for at least 6 months after getting fillers, or Botox, or any other invasive procedure. Rather not risk it, as there could be adverse consequences. After all, this is your face we are talking about here! Consult a qualified medical practitioner, if in doubt.

Q: Due to time constraints, should I resort to the 10 point shortened version of your program under the heading "Facial Exercises – A Shortened Version For Those Pressed For Time"?
A: You can, but remember that the shortened version is like cheating yourself! You will not get the full benefits and rapidity of age-regression that you would have, if you do all the 20 points. Wrinkles and baggy skin will take more time to improve upon, simply because you will be making less effort. So, please try to perform the 20 points as often as possible. Face toning workouts are based on the principle of "What you put in, you get out".

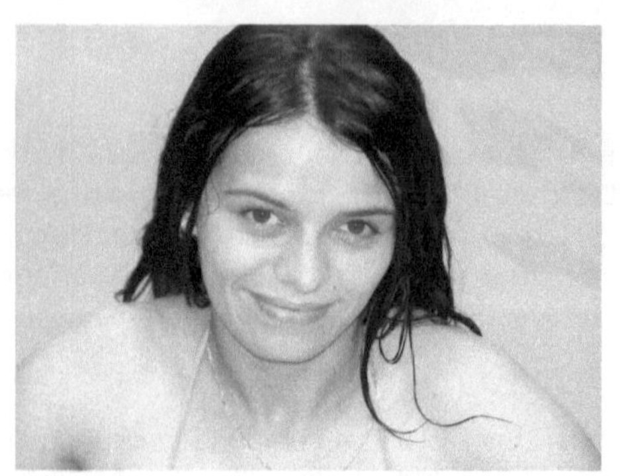

4.5. 21 Additional Ways To Keep Your Skin Young And Glowing

1. Drink plenty of water, or natural sugar-free fruit juices, every day. Toxins are flushed out in the urine. A large proportion of skin cells are made up of water, so you need to replenish any lost moisture by drinking the right liquids, at regular intervals during the day. This keeps the skin adequately hydrated. Avoid, or limit coffee and sodas if you can, as these can induce long term harm to the skin and your health.

2. Eat plenty of fiber. By consuming oats, cereals, fresh fruit and vegetables, your bowel movements will become more regular. Constipation leads to tiredness, stress, accumulation of toxins, and other complications which adversely affect the skin. Fiber in your diet keeps the body functions in balance. This boosts a healthier, more glowing skin.

3. Drink ONE WINE GLASS of dark red wine daily. The darker the red, the better. The pip and skin of the red grape is extremely rich in antioxidants, which act as a defense against free radicals such as smoke, carbon dioxide, etc. The higher your antioxidant levels, the longer the time your skin will remain looking and feeling young. Refrain from ingesting more than one glass of wine per day, as this can have an adverse effect on your skin and your liver, due to the alcohol content in the wine.

4. Take an oral Vitamin A supplement. Vitamin A is the friend of your skin. Benefits include aiding anti-aging skin care and combating acne, stretch marks, eczema, menstruation complications, urinary tract problems, wounds, infections, sinusitis, and many more. Excess Vitamin A is not excreted in the urine, like Vitamin C and the B Vitamin group, so please be cautious not to ingest too much, as there can be some nasty side-effects. Never exceed the RDA (Recommended Daily Allowance) on the bottle, or ignore the advice of a medical practitioner.

5. Take an oral Vitamin C supplement. Vitamin C plays an essential part in the incorporation of proline in collagen, and also boosts elastin (The stretchiness of the skin). This keeps wrinkles and saggy skin at bay.

6. Take an oral Vitamin E supplement. Owing to its high antioxidant content, Vitamin E is vital in protecting skin cells from ultra violet light, pollution, drugs, and other elements that produce cell damaging free radicals. It also regulates Vitamin A in the body, which is important for healthy skin.

7. Take an oral Vitamin B complex supplement. Studies have proven that Vitamin B is essential when it comes to resisting the effects of aging. Certain derivatives of Vitamin B (e.g. niacin and nicotinamide), are known to improve the ability of the epidermis (the uppermost layer of the skin) to retain moisture.

8. Take an oral Vitamin K supplement. Vitamin K is very important for protecting skin elasticity, and can prevent the skin from aging and developing wrinkles. Studies have shown that people who experience exaggerated wrinkling earlier than people of similar age, seem

to have a substantial shortage of Vitamin K in their bodies. Vitamin K is also known to fade dark circles under the eyes.

9. Take an oral Zinc supplement. Zinc is crucial for collagen production and elastin synthesis. It is required for DNA, skin damage and sunburn repair, and is an excellent medium for cell division and regrowth.

10. Take an oral Selenium supplement. Selenium assists in cell growth and reproduction, combats skin cancer and repairs damage from too much sun exposure.

11. Take an oral Copper supplement. This mineral stimulates melanin skin pigment and elastin, which prevents wrinkles.

12. Essential fatty acids (EFA's) are essential for healthy skin maintenance, especially Omega 3 and Omega 6. Through both topical application and oral consumption, they help to maintain cell structure, thereby keeping skin moisturized, smooth, and healthy. EFA's have also been known to have an anti-inflammatory effect on the skin, providing a level of relief from symptoms associated with eczema.

13. Do not bask in the sun. UVA and UVB rays contribute to premature aging, cause wrinkles, sun damage, and cancer. Over the years, due to the ozone layer thinning, even short exposure to the sun can be damaging to the skin. Rather use spray tanning, or a water-soluble bronzer to get those enviable stares!

14. Eat more leafy green vegetables and fresh fruit. It is suggested by many nutritionists that 3 different vegetables, and 3 assorted fruit types (consumed daily) are good for the skin, and for maintaining overall health.

15. Try to sleep for at least eight hours every night. Sleep is very good for the skin, and helps treat stress marks, dark eye rings, and wrinkles on the face and neck.

16. Keep base and makeup on your face to a minimum. Makeup dries and clogs the skin pores on the face and neck, thereby causing more damage than good in the long run. Short term beauty goals can cause wrinkles and accelerate aging symptoms on the face and neck, later on in life.

17. Refrain from using regular body soap to clean your face and neck. I only use a wet face cloth soaked in clean, warm water to wash my face. I thoroughly scrub my face once a day to exfoliate dead skin cells. You can also use a moisturizing soap such as Dove (Please Google it for availability in your country), and an exfoliator purchased from your local drugstore, or supermarket, to cleanse your face and neck.

18. Apply an unscented face cream on your face and neck twice a day. I prefer the Nivea Body Moisturizer for dry skin with almond oil. It is extremely rich in protein, and is one of the

best lotions to nourish and rejuvenate the skin, while performing face exercises. Do not be put off with the word "Body", as it works wonders for the face and neck!

19. Reduce stress in your life. This is often easier said than done! The skin is the body's largest organ. Stress is one of the chief contributors to wrinkles and face sag, which results in premature aging. Emotional or mental trauma can cause you to screw up your face, frown, or pout. Constant muscular contractions in the upper face eventually become permanent frown lines and wrinkles. Relaxation techniques, like the ones taught in this book (e.g. steady breathing, relaxing the shoulders), will help you to minimize stress, and relax the facial muscles and skin. Do what works for you to take the load off, such as listening to soothing music, taking a stroll in the moonlight, enjoying the company of friends, or burning incense. Relaxing for short periods during the day, can yield benefits to the skin.

20. Curb, or stop smoking altogether if you can. Smoking adversely affects the epidermis, by making it thin and dry, over time. The tar in cigarettes speeds up the production of free radicals, which are one of the skin's primary enemies. Every time you smoke, you suffocate the skin. Think of cigarettes as "wrinkle food". Lines and creases are known to manifest quicker on the face of smokers, as opposed to non-smokers of the same age.

21. Exercise as much as possible. This enhances the flow of oxygen and nutrients to the skin. It increases overall blood circulation, and is good for the heart. Exercise is known to slow down the aging process.

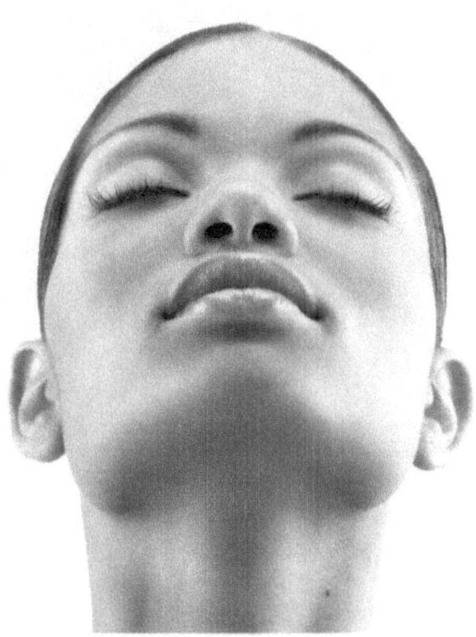

4.6. Afterword

The rest is up to you. If you adhere to the directions of this program you - your friends, and family will definitely notice a drastic improvement in your face. After the first month of diligently applying facial exercises, go into maintenance mode - by doing them at least 2-3 times a week. If you fail to do this upkeep, you could risk undoing all the excellent progress you have made with the program.

Before you start the face workouts, may I suggest you get a before and after picture taken of your face and neck. After 30 days of implementing the program, snap another photo using the same background, and possibly the same outfit. Compare the pictures. I bet you will be amazed at the difference. I would love to see your photos, so if you do get the time, please email them to me with a short note of your facial workout experience, derived from Facial Regeneration Exercises.

Feel free to contact me at naturalfacelift@yahoo.com with any questions.

I look forward to hearing from you.

Enjoy the program, and I wish you luck in your age-regression endeavors!

Love to you all.

Wendy Wilken

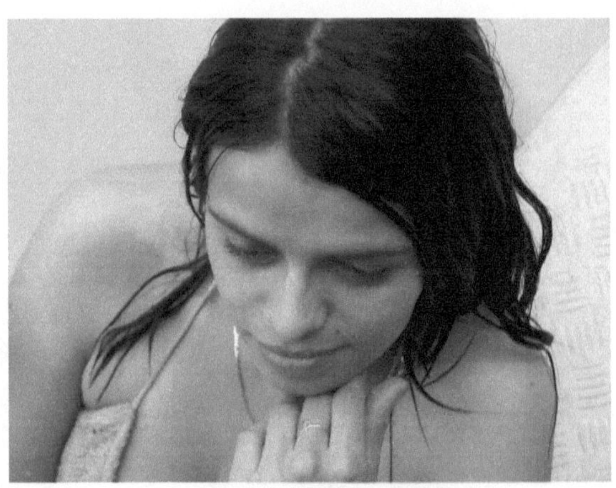

5. OTHER BOOKS AND LINKS BY THE SAME AUTHOR

Other Kindle And Soft Cover Books By the Authors:

Book 1 Of 5 Of The "Be Here Now" Addiction Kindle & Soft Cover Book Series

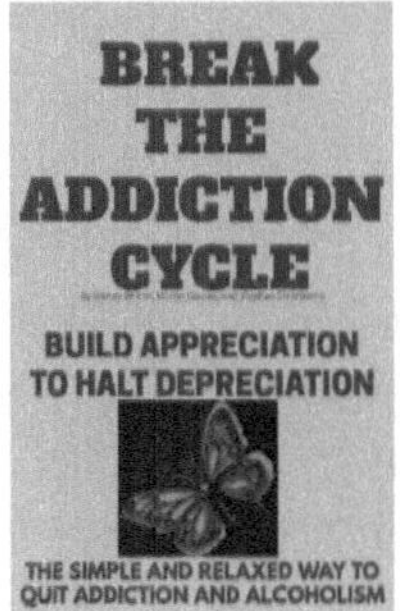

BREAK THE ADDICTION CYCLE – BUILD APPRECIATION TO HALT DEPRECIATION

You are NOT WIRED to fight your cravings for alcohol, substances, or an addictive action that GIVES YOU EMOTIONAL REWARDS. That is why AA and Rehab have such low success rates.

Lack of self-worth is the common thread that locks you in an alcohol abuse or addiction cycle. NEVER BATTLE alcoholism or addiction head-on, because you are targeting the symptoms instead of the root cause. You should only MODIFY A FEW MINOR DAILY LIFESTYLE HABITS which will build self-worth exponentially - and alcoholism/addiction falls away quickly, and effortlessly.

Stop fighting the symptoms – treat the CAUSE!

It only takes a few days - No self-discipline or battling against your cravings is needed!

Features Of This Program:
- Learn the reasons why alcoholism and addiction is not a disease but an APPARATUS
- The addiction algorithm revealed! - Discover how to flip off its switches in the correct way
- How nature can be harnessed to beat alcohol abuse and addiction
- Simple ways to build gratitude to instantly reverse all decay in your life and cure addiction
- Kick your bad habits quickly - A way to neutralize all negatives in your life
- Learn the "Shoebox" method to stop alcoholism and addiction without effort or fear
- Learn 4 magic words that rapidly change your life and dismantles your addiction apparatus
- Discover why building self-worth is the key to eradicate alcoholism and addiction
- How small daily lifestyle modifications weaken your cravings and break your binge cycles
- How to quit your addiction by harnessing nature's laws and applying gratitude in your life
- How to apply mind magnetism with "The Law Of Attraction" to end addiction
- How to use gravitational pull with "The Law Of Attraction" to halt alcoholism and addiction

Benefits Of This Program:

- A simple, easy-to-apply, relaxed approach to stop cravings, halt drinking, and quit addiction
- Written by former alcoholics and addicts who understand the TRUE DYNAMICS of addiction
- This process treats alcoholism and all forms of addiction AS AN APPARATUS, not a disease
- Exit addiction the same way you entered it - By having fun, without intention, harmoniously
- Beats all conventional alcohol abuse and addiction recovery methods
- Halt and recover from addiction alone - No need for self-help groups or other people
- The FUN way to get rid of addiction! Enjoy dismantling your addiction apparatus!
- Our approach is: You are NOT AN ADDICT, you are NOT BROKEN - You are simply fixated
- Alter a few variables in your addiction algorithm to spring free from the mind trap
- Works QUICKLY and effectively once you apply these principles to overcome your addiction
- Not only recover from alcoholism or addiction - All areas of your life will overflow with success!
- This program gets to the point quickly, without waffle or unnecessary page fillers
- NO self-discipline, no effort, no work required to cure alcohol abuse and addiction
- NO need to tackle your addiction directly - Simply make some small daily lifestyle adjustments
- NO need for constant affirmations that you are an alcoholic or addict to yourself or others
- NO uphill battle, no fight, no self-control required against cravings - Nature does it all for you!
- NO religious leaning involved - Inclusive of all beliefs and non-beliefs
- NO groveling for forgiveness to those whom you have wronged - Clean slate, a fresh start!
- NO force, no fear, no judgments to stop your addictive behavior - This is a very smooth process

The Martin Gouws "Be Here Now" program is very effective to overcome all kinds of addiction and compulsive behavior: alcoholism, substance and drug abuse, food addiction, sex addiction, pornography addiction, opioid addiction, prescription drug addiction, compulsive gambling, aggression and anger issues, kleptomania, smoking and nicotine addiction, social media addiction, texting addiction, work addiction, and caffeine addiction.

BREAK THE ADDICTION CYCLE – BUILD APPRECIATION TO HALT DEPRECIATION

Book 2 Of 5 Of The "Be Here Now" Addiction Kindle & Soft Cover Book Series

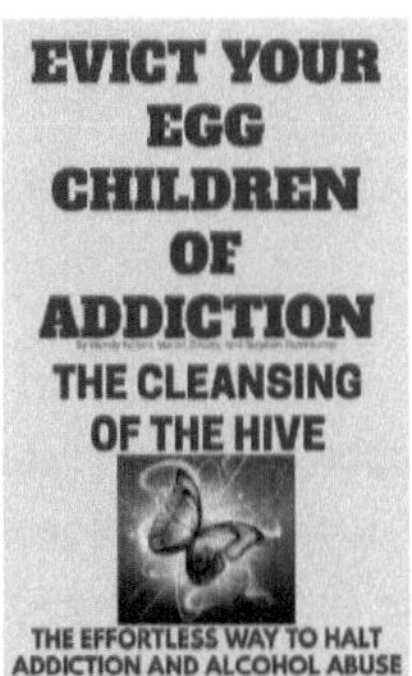

EVICT YOUR EGG CHILDREN OF ADDICTION – THE CLEANSING OF THE HIVE

You are NOT WIRED to fight your cravings for alcohol, substances, or an addictive action that GIVES YOU EMOTIONAL REWARDS. That is why AA and Rehab have such low success rates.

You unknowingly live in a "Hive" with 5 million of your egg children (skin particles and fingerprint oils) in your home. Each of them comprises your DNA that emits a continuous and subtle alcoholism or addiction sound frequency and scent that your subconscious mind is constantly receiving. This locks you in addiction. Modify these odors and frequencies in your home, and alcoholism/addiction falls away quickly, and effortlessly.

Stop fighting the symptoms – treat the CAUSE!

It only takes a few days - No self-discipline or battling against your cravings is needed!

Features Of This Program:
- Learn about the components of your addiction apparatus and how it functions like an algorithm
- How the 2 you's interact in your unique addiction apparatus and lock you in addiction
- The hidden enemy that lives with you REVEALED! - How to alter your addiction signature
- Why you are unwittingly transporting your addiction wherever you go and how to stop this
- Revealed: The 4 "Hive" aspects of addiction and how to conquer them with a few minor tweaks
- How to change 2 of your senses from foe to friend to overcome alcoholism and addiction
- Why the "Throw The Baby Out With The Bathwater" mindset is so effective to quit addiction
- How to INSTANTLY BLOCK YOUR CRAVINGS with a simple drugstore gel
- Learn 20 killer tips to modify your home environment that will eradicate your addictive behavior
- Learn the secrets to change the sound frequencies and odors in your home to stop addiction

- Discover little-known everyday lifestyle changes that dissolve alcohol abuse and addiction fast
- Learn small modifications in your living and work environments to free yourself from addiction

Benefits Of This Program:
- A simple, easy-to-apply, relaxed approach to stop cravings, halt drinking, and quit addiction
- Written by former alcoholics and addicts who understand the TRUE DYNAMICS of addiction
- This process treats alcoholism and all forms of addiction AS AN APPARATUS, not a disease
- Exit addiction the same way you entered it - By having fun, without intention, harmoniously
- Beats all conventional alcohol abuse and addiction recovery methods
- Halt and recover from addiction alone - No need for self-help groups or other people
- The FUN way to get rid of addiction! Enjoy dismantling your addiction apparatus!
- Our approach is: You are NOT AN ADDICT, you are NOT BROKEN - You are simply fixated
- Alter a few variables in your addiction algorithm to spring free from the mind trap
- Works QUICKLY and effectively once you apply these principles to overcome your addiction
- Not only recover from alcoholism or addiction - All areas of your life will overflow with success!
- This program gets to the point quickly, without waffle or unnecessary page fillers
- NO self-discipline, no effort, no work required to cure alcohol abuse and addiction
- NO need to tackle your addiction directly - Simply make some small daily lifestyle adjustments
- NO need for constant affirmations that you are an alcoholic or addict to yourself or others
- NO uphill battle, no fight, no self-control required against cravings - Nature does it all for you!
- NO religious leaning involved - Inclusive of all beliefs and non-beliefs
- NO groveling for forgiveness to those whom you have wronged - Clean slate, a fresh start!
- NO force, no fear, no judgments to stop your addictive behavior - This is a very smooth process

The Martin Gouws "Be Here Now" program is very effective to overcome all kinds of addiction and compulsive behavior: alcoholism, substance and drug abuse, food addiction, sex addiction, pornography addiction, opioid addiction, prescription drug addiction, compulsive gambling, aggression and anger issues, kleptomania, smoking and nicotine addiction, social media addiction, texting addiction, work addiction, and caffeine addiction.

EVICT YOUR EGG CHILDREN OF ADDICTION – THE CLEANSING OF THE HIVE

Book 3 Of 5 Of The "Be Here Now" Addiction Kindle & Soft Cover Book Series

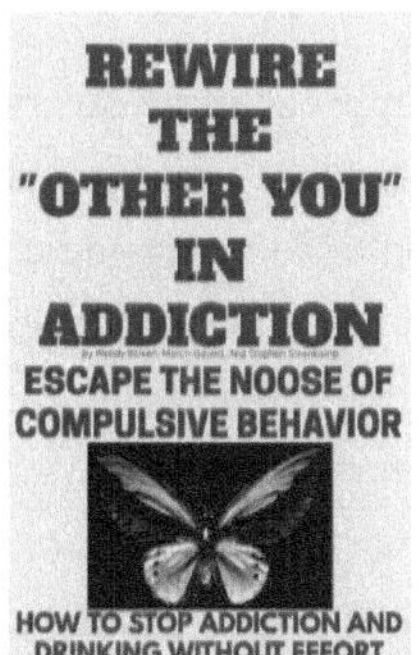

REWIRE THE "OTHER YOU" IN ADDICTION – ESCAPE THE NOOSE OF COMPULSIVE BEHAVIOR

You are NOT WIRED to fight your cravings for alcohol, substances, or an addictive action that GIVES YOU EMOTIONAL REWARDS. That is why AA and Rehab have such low success rates.

It is the hidden enemy of the "Other You" that locks you in alcoholism or addiction. You need to balance the "Other You" WITH YOUR HOME ENVIRONMENT. Simply make a few SMALL DAILY LIFESTYLE CHANGES, such as altering the subtle alcoholism or addiction odors and sound frequencies in your surroundings. This smashes your binge cycles and collapses your addiction apparatus. When you harmonize the "Other You", alcoholism/addiction falls away quickly, and effortlessly.

Stop fighting the symptoms – treat the CAUSE!

It only takes a few days - No self-discipline or battling against your cravings is needed!

Features Of This Program:
- Discover the identity of the 2 you's and how each plays a role in alcoholism and addiction
- The reason why drinking or addiction is not your fault - It is the "Other You" with addiction
- How you unwittingly built your addiction apparatus with the 2 you's
- Find out who the "Watchers" really are and why you often become paranoid during binges
- Learn 3 secrets that allow nature to cure your alcoholism or addiction smoothly for you
- How to manipulate the push-pull factors of addiction - Block your cravings with ease
- How to smash your binge cycles by changing the resonance and odors of the "Other You"
- Use 21 minor household tweaks for a new "Other You" - Naturally break down your binge cycles
- Discover how to harmoniously quit alcohol abuse and addiction by balancing the 2 you's
- Learn 3 MINIMAL daily lifestyle modifications to free you from the mind trap of addiction
- How a cheap drugstore gel INSTANTLY BLOCKS YOUR CRAVINGS! – Exit addiction with ease
- The secrets to ushering in a new higher state "Other You" free from alcoholism and addiction

Benefits Of This Program:

- A simple, easy-to-apply, relaxed approach to stop cravings, halt drinking, and quit addiction
- Written by former alcoholics and addicts who understand the TRUE DYNAMICS of addiction
- This process treats alcoholism and all forms of addiction AS AN APPARATUS, not a disease
- Exit addiction the same way you entered it - By having fun, without intention, harmoniously
- Beats all conventional alcohol abuse and addiction recovery methods
- Halt and recover from addiction alone - No need for self-help groups or other people
- The FUN way to get rid of addiction! Enjoy dismantling your addiction apparatus!
- Our approach is: You are NOT AN ADDICT, you are NOT BROKEN - You are simply fixated
- Alter a few variables in your addiction algorithm to spring free from the mind trap
- Works QUICKLY and effectively once you apply these principles to overcome your addiction
- Not only recover from alcoholism or addiction - All areas of your life will overflow with success!
- This program gets to the point quickly, without waffle or unnecessary page fillers
- NO self-discipline, no effort, no work required to cure alcohol abuse and addiction
- NO need to tackle your addiction directly - Simply make some small daily lifestyle adjustments
- NO need for constant affirmations that you are an alcoholic or addict to yourself or others
- NO uphill battle, no fight, no self-control required against cravings - Nature does it all for you!
- NO religious leaning involved - Inclusive of all beliefs and non-beliefs
- NO groveling for forgiveness to those whom you have wronged - Clean slate, a fresh start!
- NO force, no fear, no judgments to stop your addictive behavior - This is a very smooth process

The Martin Gouws "Be Here Now" program is very effective to overcome all kinds of addiction and compulsive behavior: alcoholism, substance and drug abuse, food addiction, sex addiction, pornography addiction, opioid addiction, prescription drug addiction, compulsive gambling, aggression and anger issues, kleptomania, smoking and nicotine addiction, social media addiction, texting addiction, work addiction, and caffeine addiction.

REWIRE THE "OTHER YOU" IN ADDICTION – ESCAPE THE NOOSE OF COMPULSIVE BEHAVIOR

Book 4 Of 5 Of The "Be Here Now" Addiction Kindle & Soft Cover Book Series

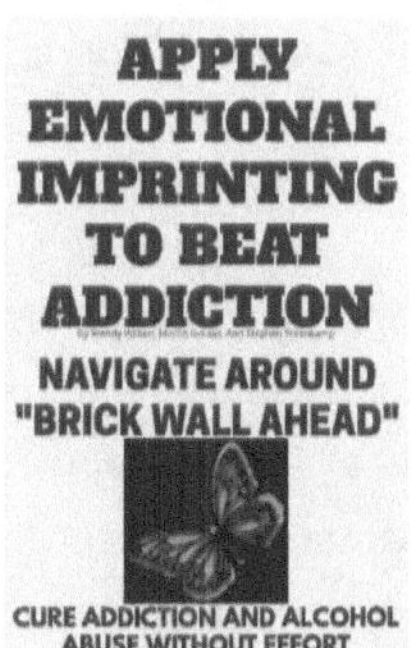# APPLY EMOTIONAL IMPRINTING TO BEAT ADDICTION – NAVIGATE AROUND "BRICK WALL AHEAD"

You are NOT WIRED to fight your cravings for alcohol, substances, or an addictive action that GIVES YOU EMOTIONAL REWARDS. That is why AA and Rehab have such low success rates.

Past bad emotions create bad memories that produce subconscious smells and subtle sound frequencies. These lock you in the mind trap of alcoholism or addiction. Alter these subtle odors and sound resonance in your living environment - and you automatically CREATE NEW HIGHER STATE EMOTIONS that remove the need for substances or addictive actions. Alcoholism/Addiction then falls away quickly, and effortlessly.

Stop fighting the symptoms – treat the CAUSE!

It only takes a few days - No self-discipline or battling against your cravings is needed!

Features Of This Program:
- How smells, memories, and bad emotions erect an APPARATUS OF ADDICTION around you
- What really makes alcoholism and addiction tick - If you know this, you WILL beat addiction!
- Learn how to crack your unique addiction algorithm to collapse your addiction apparatus
- How to switch from brain thinking to "Heart Mind" mode - Dissipate your binge cycles easily!
- Learn 3 simple principles that break down the tight circle of alcohol abuse and addiction
- How a few daily lifestyle adjustments boost your emotions and remove your cravings
- Learn the secrets of emotional imprinting and how it can be shaped to beat your addiction
- How a cheap supermarket gel HALTS YOUR CRAVINGS INSTANTLY!
- Find out why altering odors and sound frequencies in your home eradicates addiction
- End your binge cycles naturally using highly effective observation and measurement methods
- Revealed – The 2 "Laws Of Attraction" that speedily dissolve cravings and halt your addiction

- The secrets for a new circle of success - Spring free from addiction using emotional imprinting

Benefits Of This Program:
- A simple, easy-to-apply, relaxed approach to stop cravings, halt drinking, and quit addiction
- Written by former alcoholics and addicts who understand the TRUE DYNAMICS of addiction
- This process treats alcoholism and all forms of addiction AS AN APPARATUS, not a disease
- Exit addiction the same way you entered it - By having fun, without intention, harmoniously
- Beats all conventional alcohol abuse and addiction recovery methods
- Halt and recover from addiction alone - No need for self-help groups or other people
- The FUN way to get rid of addiction! Enjoy dismantling your addiction apparatus!
- Our approach is: You are NOT AN ADDICT, you are NOT BROKEN - You are simply fixated
- Alter a few variables in your addiction algorithm to spring free from the mind trap
- Works QUICKLY and effectively once you apply these principles to overcome your addiction
- Not only recover from alcoholism or addiction - All areas of your life will overflow with success!
- This program gets to the point quickly, without waffle or unnecessary page fillers
- NO self-discipline, no effort, no work required to cure alcohol abuse and addiction
- NO need to tackle your addiction directly - Simply make some small daily lifestyle adjustments
- NO need for constant affirmations that you are an alcoholic or addict to yourself or others
- NO uphill battle, no fight, no self-control required against cravings - Nature does it all for you!
- NO religious leaning involved - Inclusive of all beliefs and non-beliefs
- NO groveling for forgiveness to those whom you have wronged - Clean slate, a fresh start!
- NO force, no fear, no judgments to stop your addictive behavior - This is a very smooth process

The Martin Gouws "Be Here Now" program is very effective to overcome all kinds of addiction and compulsive behavior: alcoholism, substance and drug abuse, food addiction, sex addiction, pornography addiction, opioid addiction, prescription drug addiction, compulsive gambling, aggression and anger issues, kleptomania, smoking and nicotine addiction, social media addiction, texting addiction, work addiction, and caffeine addiction.

APPLY EMOTIONAL IMPRINTING TO BEAT ADDICTION – NAVIGATE AROUND "BRICK WALL AHEAD"

Book 5 Of 5 Of The "Be Here Now" Addiction Kindle & Soft Cover Book Series

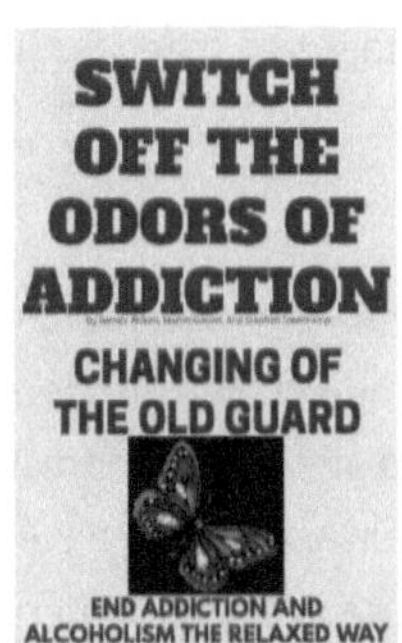

SWITCH OFF THE ODORS OF ADDICTION – CHANGING OF THE OLD GUARD

You are NOT WIRED to fight your cravings for alcohol, substances, or an addictive action that GIVES YOU EMOTIONAL REWARDS. That is why AA and Rehab have such low success rates.

Odors, memories, and "Bad Feel" emotions are closely linked. Your brain is subconsciously receiving scent traces of your alcoholism or addiction in your home, and on your personal items - which lock you in a mind trap. Make just a few MINOR DAILY LIFESTYLE ADJUSTMENTS and this will automatically alter these odors. Alcoholism/Addiction then falls away quickly, and effortlessly.

Stop fighting the symptoms – treat the CAUSE!

It only takes a few days - No self-discipline or battling against your cravings is needed!

Features Of This Program:
- Discover why you are a master builder of your own unique addiction apparatus
- How your 5 senses link to bad memories - Learn the main cause of alcoholism and addiction
- Revealed: ENEMY NUMBER ONE in addiction - The link of odors to past, present, and future
- How your home and work environments lock you in addiction - Learn 2 secrets to break free!
- Take a peek at your addiction algorithm - Learn which switches to flip to quit your addiction!
- Why you are transporting your addiction stench wherever you go - How to stop this right now
- A simple drugstore gel that BLOCKS YOUR CRAVINGS INSTANTLY! - Nobody knows this secret!
- Learn how to swap out old compulsive behavior odors and create fresh ones to quit addiction
- 19 sizzling hot tips to quickly change the smells around you! - Exit addiction with ease
- How to dismantle your addiction apparatus - Transform your worst enemy into your best friend
- Why NEW smells force you to lose interest in your vice quickly – Fast-track out of addiction!

- Discover simple daily lifestyle changes to free you from addiction and build success in your life

Benefits Of This Program:
- A simple, easy-to-apply, relaxed approach to stop cravings, halt drinking, and quit addiction
- Written by former alcoholics and addicts who understand the TRUE DYNAMICS of addiction
- This process treats alcoholism and all forms of addiction AS AN APPARATUS, not a disease
- Exit addiction the same way you entered it - By having fun, without intention, harmoniously
- Beats all conventional alcohol abuse and addiction recovery methods
- Halt and recover from addiction alone - No need for self-help groups or other people
- The FUN way to get rid of addiction! Enjoy dismantling your addiction apparatus!
- Our approach is: You are NOT AN ADDICT, you are NOT BROKEN - You are simply fixated
- Alter a few variables in your addiction algorithm to spring free from the mind trap
- Works QUICKLY and effectively once you apply these principles to overcome your addiction
- Not only recover from alcoholism or addiction - All areas of your life will overflow with success!
- This program gets to the point quickly, without waffle or unnecessary page fillers
- NO self-discipline, no effort, no work required to cure alcohol abuse and addiction
- NO need to tackle your addiction directly - Simply make some small daily lifestyle adjustments
- NO need for constant affirmations that you are an alcoholic or addict to yourself or others
- NO uphill battle, no fight, no self-control required against cravings - Nature does it all for you!
- NO religious leaning involved - Inclusive of all beliefs and non-beliefs
- NO groveling for forgiveness to those whom you have wronged - Clean slate, a fresh start!
- NO force, no fear, no judgments to stop your addictive behavior - This is a very smooth process

The Martin Gouws "Be Here Now" program is very effective to overcome all kinds of addiction and compulsive behavior: alcoholism, substance and drug abuse, food addiction, sex addiction, pornography addiction, opioid addiction, prescription drug addiction, compulsive gambling, aggression and anger issues, kleptomania, smoking and nicotine addiction, social media addiction, texting addiction, work addiction, and caffeine addiction.

SWITCH OFF THE ODORS OF ADDICTION – CHANGING OF THE OLD GUARD

All 5 Books Consolidated In One Main "Be Here Now" Addiction Kindle & Soft Cover Book Series

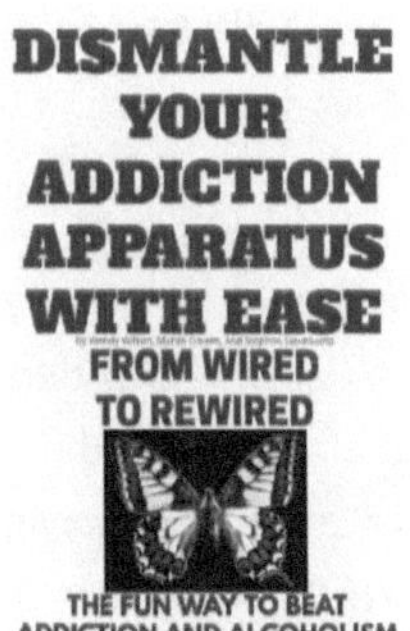

DISMANTLE YOUR ADDICTION APPARATUS WITH EASE – FROM WIRED TO REWIRED

Quit alcoholism and addiction by going with the grain of human nature, and not against it. There should be NO FIGHTING your cravings and NO SELF-CONTROL battles. Overcoming alcohol abuse and addiction is actually simple, relaxing, and loads of FUN - if you do it right! If you are trying to beat addiction any other way, then you are doing it wrong.

Stop fighting the symptoms – treat the CAUSE!

The Martin Gouws "Be Here Now" process is stress-free and easy to implement. Nature does all the work for you.

It only takes a few days - No self-discipline or battling against your cravings is needed!

Features Of This Program:
- Discover how to tap into nature's resources to halt alcoholism and addiction
- Learn the 4 elements of your addiction apparatus - Change ONE and you will beat addiction!
- Check out your unique addiction algorithm! Learn how to flip the correct switches
- The fun, easy, laidback way to end addiction - Learn how to implement "Option 3" in your life
- Meet the "Other You" who is the addict - Balance the 2 you's and addiction WILL be overcome
- Halt your binge cycles quickly with the "Shoebox" method - Break out of the addiction mind trap
- How 3 minor lifestyle changes break down binge cycles and destroys your addiction circle
- Why the truth will set you free from alcoholism and addiction - 3 questions that always yield truth
- 21 killer tips to beat your addiction by changing odors and sound frequencies in your home
- BEST KEPT SECRET REVEALED: A cheap drugstore gel that blocks your cravings INSTANTLY!
- How to fast-track out of alcohol abuse and addiction by applying emotional imprinting
- Why observation and measurement is a powerful weapon for recovery from addiction

- How to cure alcoholism and addiction with 2 powerful elements of "The Law Of Attraction"
- A dynamic way to overcome drinking and addiction with the "Birds Of A Feather" rule

Benefits Of This Program:
- A simple, easy-to-apply, relaxed approach to stop cravings, halt drinking, and quit addiction
- Written by former alcoholics and addicts who understand the TRUE DYNAMICS of addiction
- This process treats alcoholism and all forms of addiction AS AN APPARATUS, not a disease
- Exit addiction the same way you entered it - By having fun, without intention, harmoniously
- Beats all conventional alcohol abuse and addiction recovery methods
- Halt and recover from addiction alone - No need for self-help groups or other people
- The FUN way to get rid of addiction! Enjoy dismantling your addiction apparatus!
- Our approach is: You are NOT AN ADDICT, you are NOT BROKEN - You are simply fixated
- Alter a few variables in your addiction algorithm to spring free from the mind trap
- Works QUICKLY and effectively once you apply these principles to overcome your addiction
- Not only recover from alcoholism or addiction - All areas of your life will overflow with success!
- This program gets to the point quickly, without waffle or unnecessary page fillers
- NO self-discipline, no effort, no work required to cure alcohol abuse and addiction
- NO need to tackle your addiction directly - Simply make some small daily lifestyle adjustments
- NO need for constant affirmations that you are an alcoholic or addict to yourself or others
- NO uphill battle, no fight, no self-control required against cravings - Nature does it all for you!
- NO religious leaning involved - Inclusive of all beliefs and non-beliefs
- NO groveling for forgiveness to those whom you have wronged - Clean slate, a fresh start!
- NO force, no fear, no judgments to stop your addictive behavior - This is a very smooth process

The Martin Gouws "Be Here Now" program is very effective to overcome all kinds of addiction and compulsive behavior: alcoholism, substance and drug abuse, food addiction, sex addiction, pornography addiction, opioid addiction, prescription drug addiction, compulsive gambling, aggression and anger issues, kleptomania, smoking and nicotine addiction, social media addiction, texting addiction, work addiction, and caffeine addiction.

DISMANTLE YOUR ADDICTION APPARATUS WITH EASE – FROM WIRED TO REWIRED

Wendy Wilken also has 2 other publications on 2 different websites on the subject of facial exercises for men and women to look younger:

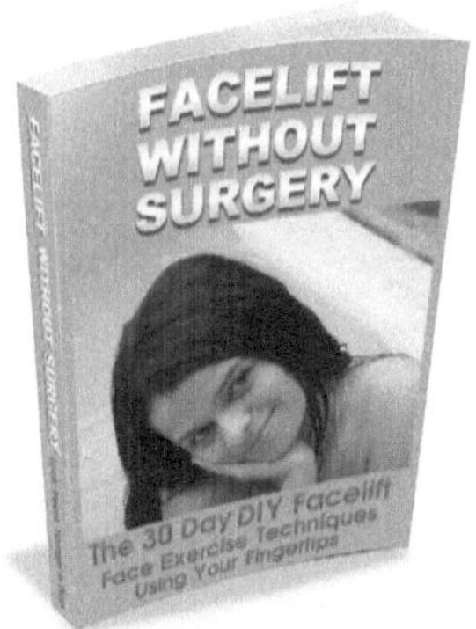

FACELIFT WITHOUT SURGERY
Facial Exercises Program By Wendy Wilken
www.facelift-without-surgery.biz

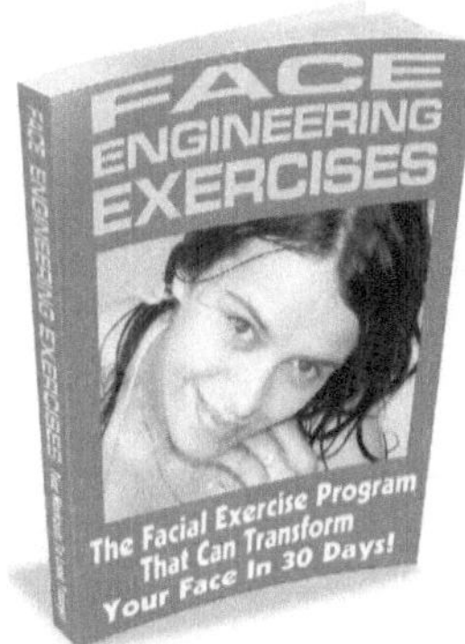

FACE ENGINEERING EXERCISES
Facial Exercises Program By Wendy Wilken
www.face-engineering-exercises.org

www.ingramcontent.com/pod-product-compliance
Lightning Source LLC
Chambersburg PA
CBHW030358280726
48655CB00019B/2320